HEALTH

INSURANCE

in America

HEALTH INSURANCE

in America

A CONSUMER'S GUIDE

2nd Edition

C.W. Conrad

Printed in the United States of America

First Printing: May 2020

ISBN: 979-8-7347-1674-8

Disclaimer: THIS GUIDE DOES NOT PROVIDE MEDICAL ADVICE. The author is not a medical professional. Always seek the advice of your physician or other qualified health provider with any questions you may have regarding a medical condition. Never disregard professional medical advice or delay in seeking it because of something you have read in this guide.

To contact the author.
email: CWConradbooks@gmail.com
Website: CWConrad-Books.com
Instagram: @CWConradbooks

CONTENTS

Part I - Introduction to Health Insurance

Part II – Choosing Your Plan

Part III – Now You've Got a Plan

Part IV – Things to Watch out For

Part V – Advanced Topics

FOREWARD

Chances are, you have had some kind of experience with health insurance in the past, and if you haven't, you probably will in the future. If you don't understand the terms and acronyms that are used, it can be confusing and frustrating to have to deal with the numerous people involved in healthcare and health insurance. To many, it's a mysterious black-box. You go see your family doctor, some things happen behind the health insurance curtain, and you get a bill.   But you never really know or understand exactly what is happening behind the scenes. Do you need to understand how it works to use it? No. But it sure is helpful. According to data from Bend Financial in a recent Forbes Magazine article:

> Confusion about health insurance is costing Americans money and preventing many from getting the care they need…… Previous research has shown that confusion about health insurance leads consumers to choose more costly coverage than they need and uncertainty about cost can cause people to delay or avoid medical care.

> Asked what element of health insurance confuses them most, 52% of respondents said figuring out what counts toward their deductible, 47% said what procedures are covered, and 47% said what constitutes in- or out-of-network care (Gordon, 2021).

> Hopefully, you never experience a health-insurance-related problem. But what if you do? Who do you call? If you manage to reach the right person, do the insurance company's answers make sense, and how do you know they have fully understood your questions or issue in

the first place? Are you able to communicate in the insurance company's language? When selecting health insurance, it can be just as confusing and frustrating. Which choice is best for you and your family? Which choices do you make after you select your insurance that will make your insurance work the best for you?

Those are all good questions. This guide is intended to give you the understanding and the tools to make smart health insurance and healthcare choices, communicate with providers and health insurance companies, and understand what you are being told throughout the process.

This is the first book of its kind, containing a complete picture of health insurance, written in a way that is easy for you, the consumer, to understand. This guide is intended to educate you about the complex world of health insurance and help you answer questions about your particular health insurance situation.

Use this guide to understand your options, and understand how to make the right decisions. But do not rely on this guide alone to dictate which choices to make. Use multiple sources if you can. You should always reach out to your insurance company, or if your employer is offering health insurance and you have questions, you should consult with your employer's HR department. If you are purchasing private health insurance, there will always be a number you can call to discuss your questions. Employers try to educate employees about the benefits they offer. But without counseling each employee, there is no guarantee the employee is making the best choices about coverage.

The information in this guide is presented in a way that makes it easy to understand, with common examples throughout. This guide touches on many topics, and is written at a high level. Some of the topics may not apply to your particular situation. If more in-depth knowledge about any of the topics is desired, this guide will give you the background you need to continue your learning journey.

Since health insurance is highly regulated by the government, the rules change often. The information in this guide is accurate as of the time of writing, but beware of changing policies. This guide provides the knowledge you need to better understand political candidates' platforms, and can help you form your own opinions as they relate to the political landscape of healthcare and health insurance.

Some of the topics in this guide are not entirely about health insurance. Even though they may not be directly related to health insurance, they are often performed by insurance companies or have a major impact on healthcare and health insurance costs. In addition, you can't discuss health insurance without discussing – in one way or another – healthcare. The healthcare decisions that we make are often dictated by the type and level of insurance coverage we have. So the two topics must be discussed together.

Whenever you see this symbol in this guide, it suggests something that you should pay attention to. Possibly things that are often confusing to consumers, leading to bad healthcare decisions, or are just items that are important to know.

Wishing you a Healthy and Happy Life!

ACKNOWLEDGMENTS

I want to acknowledge Chris and Kate for their ideas and suggestion that lead to the first edition of this book. In addition, my good friend Anthony was a technical reviewer, and I appreciate his review and feedback. Lorie came thru in a big way providing valuable insight.

Part I - Introduction to Health Insurance

CHAPTER 1

The Basics

This chapter provides an overview of health insurance and builds the foundation for all subsequent chapters of the guide. You will learn what health insurance is, the kind of expenses it pays for, how health insurance is obtained, and why it's important that it be available to everyone.

Rising Healthcare Costs

Healthcare costs in the United States are increasing at an alarming rate. According to a study from the Centers for Medicare and Medicaid Services (CMS), national health spending is projected to grow at an average annual rate of 5.4 percent from 2019-28 and reach $6.2 trillion by 2028. In 2018, out-of-pocket spending grew 2.8 percent to $375.6 billion and prescription drug spending increased 2.5 percent to $335.0 billion. (CMS.gov, Page Last Modified: 03/24/2020). Healthcare spending is placing a tremendous burden on people's personal finances. In addition to every-day healthcare costs, a long hospital stay or surgical procedure could result in hundreds of thousands of dollars in bills. There are many cases where people have had their savings and retirement completely wiped out by unexpected medical situations. Medical related bills have become the number one reason for unpaid bills being sent to collection agencies. According to a study performed by consumer finance company Credit Karma, an analysis of nearly twenty million members in the U.S. found that they have a total of forty-five billion dollars of medical debt in collections, which averages to about $2,200 of debt per member. A separate survey performed by Debt.com showed that fifty-six percent of U.S. adults had medical debt sent to collections and five percent owe more than $50,000. (Menton, 2020)

Even with health insurance, millions of American households do not have the immediate financial resources to pay their medical deductible if a large medical bill is incurred. This often leads to drawing from retirement accounts or taking loans which further deteriorates the family's financial footing. A joint study by the Kaiser Foundation and the LA Times published in 2019 found that "[f]our in ten report that their family has had either a problem paying medical bills or difficulty affording premiums or out-of-pocket medical costs, and about half say someone in their household skipped or postponed some type of medical care or prescription drugs in the past year because of the cost. Sadly, seventeen percent say they've had to make what they feel are difficult sacrifices in order to pay healthcare or insurance costs; for some, the sacrifices they report making are extreme" (Hamel, Munana, & Brodie, 2019).

When all else fails, many families are forced into bankruptcy. Vermont senator Bernie Sanders, in his 2020 presidential campaign asserted that "500,000 Americans will go bankrupt this year from medical bills". Probably an exaggeration, but you get the point.

Rather than face bankruptcy or complete liquidation of retirement funds, more-and-more people are turning to alternate funding sources such as GoFundMe. According to GoFundMe.com, they are the leader in online medical fundraising, hosting over 120 medical campaigns per year, and raising over $650 million per year.

In addition to medical expenses, the cost of some medications is ridiculously high due to the cost of research and development, marketing expenses, and "Big Pharma's" increasingly high profits. Seldom used drugs that are only used to treat rare diseases are ridiculously expensive. For instance, according to GoodRx.com, and their list of the twenty most expensive drugs in 2019, Myalept (used to treat leptin deficiency in patients with generalized lipodystrophy, a condition of abnormal fat distribution in the body) retails for $64,859 for a one-month supply, and Ravicti (used to treat urea cycle disorders, which are genetic conditions that result in high levels of ammonia in the blood) retails for $52,756 for a one-month supply. The other drugs on the list all retail for at least $30,000 per month. No one pays the retail price, but this illustrates the potential costs.

What is Health Insurance?

Risk is defined as "exposing (someone or something) to danger, harm or loss. Insurance is a tool that is used to help minimize risk. In general, if you do not have insurance, you are taking a risk. If you do not have car insurance, you are assuming you will not have an accident and you are taking a risk. If you do not have health insurance, you are risking that you will not be injured or sick. Insurance is considered risk management because you are taking some action to lessen the impact if the risk occurs.

When you have insurance (whatever kind), you have peace-of-mind that if something does occur, the impact will be minimized. The more likely you are to have an automobile accident or get sick, the bigger the risk. Insurance is a major component of managing risk.

i

> *The first U.S. insurance firm was founded in 1850. It offered insurance against injuries received during an accident. The first hospital and medical expense insurance was introduced in the 1920s.*
>
> *Did you know that Benjamin Franklin helped create the insurance industry in the United States in the eighteenth century to protect houses from loss due to fire, which was a common problem/risk at the time?*

The risk is extremely high if you do not have insurance. If you are willing to take the risk that nothing will ever happen to you requiring medical attention, or that anything that does happen will be minor in nature, then you may be willing to assume that risk.

Health insurance is a type of insurance coverage that pays for some or all of the medical expenses incurred by the person who has the insurance. We will call this person who is covered by insurance "the insured" and the entity that provides the insurance "the insurer". Health insurance can either pay a provider of medical services directly, or reimburse you for expenses you incur as a result of medical treatment. For a small fee called a "premium", you transfer some of the risk to another party by purchasing health insurance. The insurer could be a company who specializes in providing health insurance (called fully-insured coverage), or sometimes in the case of self-insurance, which you will read about later, the risk is transferred to your employer, who sponsors your health insurance plan. In either case, you share the risk with someone else. Insurance that only protects you from the cost of catastrophic health-related events, is important even if you do not have complete coverage.

Where Do You Get Health Insurance?

Most employers offer their employees health insurance as part of the benefits of being employed. Employers work with brokers to create a package of health insurance benefits, called a "plan", or "health insurance plan", to offer to their employees. The premium cost is then shared by the employer and the employee. Companies that can afford to do so, pay more of the cost of the premium, and the employee is responsible for the remainder. Most people do not realize that the twenty or thirty dollars a week that comes out of their pay is only a portion of the total premium paid for the health insurance they have. Some employers pay the entire premium and offer employees free health insurance.

You can also purchase health insurance policies from hundreds of private insurance companies. If you purchase private insurance (not through your employer), you will pay a premium to the private insurance company, and you will have a variety of plans to choose from. Many companies have websites that allow you to purchase health insurance online just like auto insurance.

The federal government operates a service that helps people shop for and enroll in affordable health insurance plans called the "marketplace" or "exchange". The health insurance marketplace gives consumers the ability to shop for health insurance plans through the health insurance marketplace website at HealthCare.gov. Some states run similar marketplaces.

What Does Health Insurance Pay For?

Every health insurance plan is different. Employers or insurance companies determine what benefits they are going to offer in what is referred to as a "plan". You can think of it as a plan to cover your medical expenses. Every plan contains a different level of benefits, meaning the plan pays a different portion of your expenses and possibly only certain kinds of expenses. When you are offered health insurance through your employer, you may or may not have choices about what plan you can select. If you do not have health insurance through your employer, you can purchase private health insurance and have nearly unlimited choices of benefit combinations. However, as with anything, the more benefits you purchase, the higher the premium.

In addition to medical insurance, most employers and private insurance companies offer dental, vision and drug coverage as well as other health-related benefits. As with medical insurance, dental, vision and drug plans have different benefits with different costs. This guide focuses on the medical and prescription drug portions of health insurance plans.

Why Do You Need Health Insurance?

If you do not have health insurance, you are putting yourself and your financial stability at risk. If you have some kind of medical problem that you know does or will require medical care, then it's a no-brainer. It will benefit you to have health insurance to pay part of your medical expenses. Health insurance puts your mind at ease. You can relax knowing that your finances are protected from being wiped out if an accident or major illness occurs.

If you look at the bigger picture. Why do we want people to have health insurance? When you have health insurance, you are more likely to go to see a physician when you are ill before your illness becomes unmanageable. Saying it another way, when you don't have health insurance, you are likely to avoid seeking medical care until it becomes unbearable. When you allow conditions to become critical before seeking care, it costs more to treat them, the bills are larger, and the results could be catastrophic.

For example:

A woman who had flu-like symptoms, could not afford to see a doctor, and died at home.

A man who died due to an untreated liver disease, an illness that went undiagnosed until a few weeks before his death. It was only discovered when he went to the emergency room because he was unable to afford to see a doctor due to lack of insurance coverage and inability to afford treatment out of pocket.

A woman in Pennsylvania was diagnosed with oral cancer. She has had surgery to remove the cancer, but is supposed to receive annual scans to monitor the cancer. Her doctor warned her that it is an aggressive form of cancer that will come back someday and she needs to stay on top of it. She hasn't had a scan in four years because she cannot afford it.

A woman in New Jersey was diagnosed with stage three ovarian cancer. She was laid off and did not have insurance. She struggled to pay for coverage through Cobra, plus copays and medical debt not covered by insurance. The bills kept coming in. She decided to stop receiving medical treatment due to the rising costs and debt, and died a few months later.

Source: (Sainato, 2020)

In 2009 Harvard Medical School and Cambridge Health Alliance did a study published in the American Journal of Public Health. This study concluded that [there was a] forty percent increased risk of death among the uninsured. (equating to 44,789 excess deaths annually) (Obamacarefacts.com, 2015 updated 2017)

Because there are no network discounts, the bills often go unpaid. Hospitals end up providing millions of dollars of uncompensated services every year. To recoup the money they lose, hospitals and other providers are forced to charge more for their services. Thus, contributing to the already high cost of healthcare and insurance. According to a 2021 report from the American Hospital Association, hospitals of all types have provided more than $660 billion in uncompensated care to patients since the year 2000.

> *Emergency rooms are required to treat people with emergency health conditions regardless of whether they have insurance or the financial means to pay or not because of the 1986 legislation called the Emergency Medical Treatment and Labor Act (EMTALA). So, they cannot turn away emergencies even if they want to.*

The federal government provides some funding to nonprofit hospitals to offset some of the cost of unpaid bills, which takes money away from other federal programs or simply results in increased taxes. When uninsured people are faced with unexpectedly high medical bills, it can create financial chaos in their lives, other bills go unpaid, and it hurts other areas of society. This is recognized by the federal and states governments. Many states have laws requiring people to have health insurance or face fines or tax penalties.

Part of the Affordable Care Act that you will read about later in this guide required everyone to have health insurance or face a tax penalty. But that requirement was struck down by the courts as unconstitutional in 2018.

CHAPTER 2

How Health Insurance Works

In this chapter, you will learn about the components of a health insurance plan and many of the people involved who work together to make your health insurance work.

Multiple People Are Involved

When you seek medical attention, whether it is in a hospital, a doctor's office, an urgent care facility, or a lab, insurers refer to the people who provide the service(s) as "providers", regardless of the medical service they provide. In some cases, a hospital or doctor's office is considered the provider instead of a person.

When you have health insurance, you are given an ID card that contains all of the health insurance information a provider needs to know about your insurance if you seek medical care from them. If you look at your medical ID card, you might wonder, "Who are all these people?" You might see an administrator, a network, a pharmacy benefit manager or Rx provider, a dental carrier, a vision carrier, a travel network, or an out of network wrap, as well as a utilization review vendor, a healthcare management vendor, or any combination of these entities.

Healthcare, and health insurance are complex, and this complexity often translates into multiple people and multiple organizations being involved in your care. Many will argue that this is part of the reason that healthcare and health insurance are so expensive. Your health insurance ID card contains a lot of important information about your plan, and who all the players are. It is important that you protect this card, and be able to show it (either the actual card or a virtual card on a smart phone) to any provider from whom you obtain medical services.

To have a complete understanding of the health insurance landscape, you should understand some of the different entities that could be involved. The entities listed below are the most common, but there could be others depending on the particulars of your plan. Some of these people or groups of people interact directly with you, while others you will never see as they interact only with one another behind the scene. Some of these entities are discussed in more detail later in this guide but are summarized here as an introduction, to aid in understanding during the first few chapters of this guide.

Network or Provider Network

One of the things that affect the price you pay for healthcare, and the amount that your insurance plan covers is provider networks. A provider network is a group of doctors or hospitals and other types of providers who have signed contracts with a network, to accept negotiated (discounted) rates for their services. Some of the more well-known networks are Blue Cross, United Healthcare, Cigna, and Aetna. Often referred to by the acronym BUCA. A network is often referred to as a preferred provider organization (PPO).

Your health insurance plan may be structured in a way that makes providers who are members of the network the preferred option for services because their rates will be less than those of nonmember providers. Providers who are members of the network are called in-network, or participating providers. The providers are contracted with the network, and then your plan is contracted with the network as well, which gives you access to the discounted rates of the participating providers. Out-of-network providers have not agreed to provide services at discounted rates. Therefore, their services will cost more, and your health insurance plan will likely pay less.

Sometimes people confuse the network with the administrator who performs the administrative functions for your health insurance plan. For example, a company like Cigna or Aetna could be the administrator, the network, or both. The question you need answered is, "who do I call if I have a problem or a question?" Your ID card will have the number to call for customer service which will connect you with the right people to answer your health insurance plan questions. The customer service function could be performed by the administrator or the network, or someone altogether different.

Administrator or Third-Party Administrator (TPA)

The administrator is the entity that pays claims. The administrator is sometimes completely separate from the network. The benefits administrator, third party administrator, or simply administrator is responsible for processing claims, and making payments to providers. Some administrators perform *only* those functions. Some Administrators perform those functions and also have other roles such as customer service.

i

> *If Cigna (for example) is the provider network your plan has a contract with, but your insurance has a third-party-administrator providing administration services, and you call Cigna, they will tell you that you are not insured with them. That's not a good feeling when you think you have no insurance.*

Pharmacy Benefit Manager (PBM)

One of the items you will most likely see on your medical ID card is the pharmacy benefit manager. Prescription drugs are often the most widely used benefit and, in many cases, the costliest. Prescription drug administration is very complex. So specialty companies were created to administer the pharmacy or prescription benefits exclusively. These specialty companies are called pharmacy benefits managers. The pharmacy benefits could be administered by the network, or in even rarer cases the administrator. But it is usually handled by a separate company that specializes in pharmacy benefits. It is worth noting that many PBMs also have retail pharmacies. CVS Caremark, Rite Aid, Walgreens operate as PBMs and also have a network of retail pharmacies.

Utilization Review Vendor

Utilization review (UR) is the process used to determine if a procedure, treatment, or medication is medically necessary. This process is performed by the UR vendor. The utilization review or utilization management vendor could be the same as the administrator. But this function is usually performed by the network, or a separate company who specializes in utilization management. The role of the utilization review vendor is to help save costs by making sure that the medical procedures that insured people are having are medically necessary. You will learn about this process in the section on preauthorization.

Healthcare Management Vendor

Everyone knows that one way to reduce healthcare costs is to ensure that people remain healthy and have minimal interaction with the healthcare system. It is also known that helping people manage the illnesses they already have will result in lower healthcare costs. Healthcare management (which can also be performed by the administrator or network) involves programs designed to keep people in good health and not need medical services. It also involves programs designed to help people manage their chronic illnesses like diabetes and heart disease. These programs help people find the right treatment options, make sure that they are following through with treatment plans, and taking medications as prescribed, and so on. This has recently become a marketing tool for some insurance companies. You will see many commercials advertising this role where nurses or other trained healthcare professionals visit people in their homes to assist with their healthcare, medications and other needs.

Wrap and Travel Networks.

Large provider networks like Cigna, Aetna, and Blue Cross have a large national footprint, with participating providers throughout the country. If you are traveling for business, or on vacation, you should be able to find a participating provider no matter where you are. But what if your health insurance plan is part of a smaller network? Some smaller networks only have participating providers in a small regional area. If your health insurance plan has one of these networks, and you find yourself needing medical care while traveling, you may not be able to find a participating provider. Or even if you have one of the larger networks, you may have an emergency that prevents you from obtaining services from one of the participating network providers. That does not mean you will have to pay the full price for the services or that your insurance will not cover anything.

Some health insurance plans also work with a secondary network called a "wrap" or "travel network". This may be a national network that also has contracts with many providers or could also be a third party who simply negotiates rates on behalf of the insurance plan. The wrap networks are skilled at negotiating, and providers will often negotiate rates rather than take a chance of not getting paid at all. These networks are often referred to as "complementary" networks because they complement or work with your primary network.

Cost Sharing

Health insurance plans are often grouped by how the costs are shared between the insured, and whoever is financially responsible for paying claims. They may also be grouped by the kind of providers or healthcare professionals or facilities that can be used. The types of plans are discussed in chapter 3. Before discussing the different types of plans, you must understand a few basic concepts of health insurance cost sharing.

The amount of money you pay to be part of a health insurance plan is called a premium. This premium is paid to someone who either directly or indirectly is financially responsible for paying your healthcare-related claims. This could be your employer or an insurance company. That entity will be referred to as the insurer, and the person who is covered by the insurance will be referred to as the insured. The premiums in health insurance are conceptually the same as any other type of insurance. Your premium is partly based on everyone else who shares your insurance, their expected claims, your previous claims, and a history of actual claims incurred by others insured by the same insurer. Those who hardly ever need medical care pay partially for those who do.

The amount the insurer expects to payout for your insurance plan's claims is based on the benefits the plan provides. And as such, the amount of premium they need to collect is also based on that calculation. A plan that covers many items will have a higher premium than a plan that covers fewer items.

Deductible:

Unless you have top-of-the-line health insurance, your plan requires that in addition to premiums you pay a portion of your healthcare costs. Usually, during the beginning of the benefit period or plan year (which usually begins in January), the burden is on you to pay the majority, with the insurer paying less. This reduces the risk that the insurer has in case you only require minimal care. This is called the plan's deductible.

The deductible is the amount you pay before the insurer begins sharing the cost. Auto insurance and homeowner's insurance have deductibles as well. Claims against those kinds of policies are usually large, and the deductible is a small portion of the loss, but the concept is the same. The insured is responsible for paying the deductible before the insurer will begin to pay anything. In health insurance, it's the same concept, except the claims are usually smaller in comparison, and it usually takes several smaller claims to cover the deductible amount.

You are responsible for paying one hundred percent of the costs until the deductible is met. If your car is damaged and you file a claim with your insurance company where your policy has a $500 deductible, then you are responsible for paying one hundred percent of the first $500 before the insurance company is responsible for anything. Insurance plans will have a deductible amount specified that is a total amount to be fulfilled throughout the policy period. You can think of it as a bucket of money.

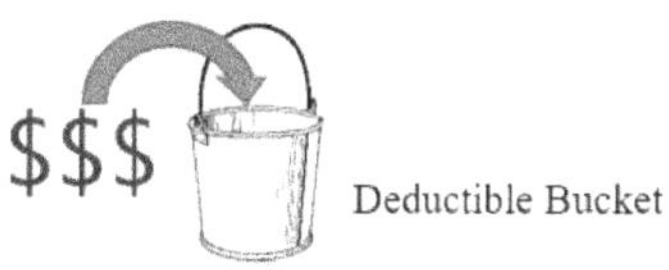

Deductible Bucket

The higher the deductible, the bigger the bucket. When the bucket is filled up, then you begin to be responsible for less of your healthcare costs and the insurer is responsible for more. When you go to a provider, whatever portion of the charges that you are responsible for is put into the deductible bucket. When the bucket is full, or the amount specified in the plan is met, then the cost sharing between you and the insurer switches to the insurer paying the majority of the cost of your medical care.

i

> *When you start a new plan year, the buckets get emptied. Regardless of how full your buckets were, you start out with empty buckets in the new plan year, and cost sharing shifts back to you.* So your out of pocket healthcare costs will usually be higher in the beginning of the year.

It states above that the insured or the insurer is responsible for the "majority" of charges. This is because before the deductible bucket is full, the government requires the insurer to pay for certain things, and even after the bucket is full, there are usually some things that you will continue to be responsible for paying. If you ever see the words "not subject to deductible" or "deductible waived", that means that the insurer pays this benefit amount even before your deductible bucket is full. The downside is, the amount of the charge is not added to your deductible bucket.

Coinsurance

After the deductible is met (the deductible bucket is full), the concept of coinsurance comes into play. Coinsurance applies during the period of cost sharing between you and the insurer. This is usually specified as a percentage in health insurance plans. It is the portion of charges that you are responsible for after the deductible bucket is filled. Coinsurance could refer to the percentage, or the period of time, (i.e. the period after the deductible is met [coinsurance period]).

For example, if you have to go to the emergency room, your plan may say there is twenty percent coinsurance. Assuming you have met your deductible amount, this means you are responsible for paying twenty percent of the total cost, and the insurer will pay the remaining eighty percent. If you have not yet met your deductible, then you will be responsible for the entire charge until the deductible bucket is filled, and *then* you will only be responsible for the coinsurance of twenty percent of the remaining amount.

Out-of-Pocket (OOP)

The out-of-pocket amount, is another bucket in health insurance plans that specifies the *total* of all expenses that you will need to pay in a policy period. The out-of-pocket limit or out-of-pocket maximum will be higher than the deductible. As the deductible bucket is filling, the OOP bucket is filling at the same time. After the deductible bucket is full and it will not hold any additional money, the costs you incur will *only* go into the OOP bucket. After the OOP bucket is full, the insurer will begin paying all expenses incurred as part of the plan. Some things do not get put into that OOP bucket, but they are very few and they are specified in the plan. After the OOP bucket is full, the coinsurance no longer applies (the coinsurance period is complete) and the insurer is responsible for one hundred percent of your medical costs.

Every plan is different, so you need to review and understand the actual plan documents for the plan you are in.

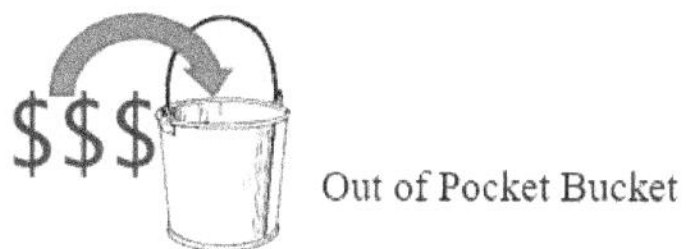

Out of Pocket Bucket

Copay

One of the ways that costs are shared between you and the insurer is called a copay. A health insurance plan will often have specific copay amounts for doctor's office visits, visits to specialists, or other specific services. For example, you may have a twenty-dollar copay for your family doctor and a thirty-dollar copay for specialists. This is the amount that you pay at the time of service with the remainder usually paid by the insurer. Lower copays, encourage you to visit your family doctor regularly rather than waiting until small problems become large health concerns because you are waiting until your deductible bucket is full. Copays do not usually get added to the deductible or OOP buckets.

i

> ## FAMILY COVERAGE
>
> *If your plan includes coverage for other family members such as your spouse or your children, then in addition to your "individual" deductible and OOP buckets, there will be family deductible and OOP buckets that are larger than the individual buckets. The family buckets get filled with charges incurred by all family members on the plan.*
>
> *Usually, you are only required to fill the individual OR the family deductible bucket before the coinsurance period begins for you. If the family bucket is filled, the entire family moves into the coinsurance period regardless of how full each person's individual bucket is. But sometimes, the family bucket must be filled before ANYONE can move to the coinsurance period.*

Review:

Here are some excerpts from an actual plan. There is a list after the graphics that contain important points regarding this plan. All examples are based on benefits for "in-network" (as opposed to "out-of-network") providers and "individual" (as opposed to "family") coverage.

		(You will pay the least)	
	Primary care visit to treat an injury or illness	20% coinsurance	5
	Specialist visit	20% coinsurance	5
If you visit a health care provider's office or clinic	Preventive care/screening/ immunization	$20 co-pay, then 100%* (Office visit only)	N
	Diagnostic test (x-ray, blood		

What is the overall <u>deductible</u>**?**	For <u>network providers</u> $650 individual / $1,250 family; for <u>out-of-network providers</u> $1,225 individual / $2,425 family
Are there services covered before you meet your <u>deductible</u>?	Yes. <u>Preventive care</u> and second surgical opinions are covered before you meet your <u>deductible</u>.

What is the <u>out-of-pocket limit</u> for this <u>plan</u>?	For <u>network providers</u> $1,000 individual / $2,000 family; for <u>out-of-network providers</u> $25,000 individual / $50,000 family
What is not included in the <u>out-of-pocket limit</u>?	<u>Premiums</u>, deductibles, co-pays, penalties, <u>balance-billing</u> charges, and health care this <u>plan</u> doesn't cover.

- If you see a provider for a routine physical exam (preventative care), you will pay a twenty-dollar copay, and the insurance will pay the remainder. (The twenty dollars *does not* go into the deductible bucket or the OOP bucket).

- If you see a provider and you are sick, and your deductible bucket is not full, you will pay one hundred percent of the charge and the entire amount will go into your deductible and OOP buckets. If your deductible bucket IS full, then you will pay twenty percent of the charge and the insurer will pay the remaining eighty percent, and the twenty percent that you pay will go into the OOP bucket.

- The deductible bucket size is $650. Once the bucket contains $650 of charges, the coinsurance will begin to apply.

- The out-of-pocket maximum is $1,000, which means that you will not need to pay more than $1,000 out of your pocket for medical expenses.

There are a lot of moving parts, and a lot of entities involved, and everything has to work together perfectly for this process to be successful, although as you will see it often fails. You need to give the provider's office correct and current information about your insurance (usually your ID card). The provider's office needs to interpret your insurance correctly and charge you the correct amount if you have a copay. The provider's office needs to put all the correct codes on the claim. The provider's office needs to send the claim to the correct place. The administrator needs to process the claim by following the benefits in your plan.   If the provider does not use the correct code on your claim, then the administrator may process the claim and misinterpret what charges go in what buckets, or they could deny the claim altogether and you will receive a bill for the full amount from the provider.

Part II – Choosing Your Plan

CHAPTER 3

Medical Plan Types

Health insurance plans come in an almost limitless combination and configuration of benefits. But there are a few basic categories of plans that share common characteristics and costs. In this chapter you will learn about the different categories of plans and some of their characteristics.

The most common types of plans today are preferred provider organization plans and high deductible health plans.

Preferred Provider Organization (PPO) Plans

A PPO plan gives you access to a network of healthcare providers and medical facilities at a reduced cost. You can choose your provider as long as they are part of the network, you don't need a referral from your primary care physician to see a specialist, and you'll also likely pay smaller copays to see specialists as opposed to other plans. Because you pay lower in-network costs, premiums for these kinds of plans tend to be higher than some of the other plan alternatives. These plans can be structured with almost any deductible and out-of-pocket limits as long as they meet the guidelines established by the government.

If you get sick while on vacation, you may not have access to in-network providers. Or, you may prefer to see a specific provider who is not in your network. Some health insurance plans pay reduced benefits for services rendered by out-of-network providers. Some provide no benefit at all for services you receive out-of-network. You are usually responsible for all the charges not paid by the health insurance plan. Many people who do not completely understand their plans and benefits do not find this out until it is too late.

Medical Event	Services You May Need	Network Provider (You will pay the least)	Out-of-Network Provider (You will pay the most)
If you visit a health care provider's office or clinic	Primary care visit to treat an injury or illness	20% coinsurance	50% coinsurance
	Specialist visit	20% coinsurance	50% coinsurance
	Preventive care/screening/ immunization	$20 co-pay, then 100%* (Office visit only)	Not Covered

Using the same plan example from before, you see that the benefit for an out of network provider is fifty percent coinsurance instead of twenty percent. So that is only fifty percent of most-likely higher, non-discounted charges. And if you see an out-of-network provider for a preventative/well visit, this particular plan will not pay anything. When your employer is the one offering the health insurance, they want to minimize costs to themselves and to their employees. So, they usually build plans that make it much less costly to see an in-network provider, and hope this encourages you to be selective about the providers you use.

High Deductible Health Plan (HDHP)

A high deductible health plan (HDHP) is a kind of PPO plan with a higher deductible than the other plan types. These plans offer a much lower premium in return for your cost-sharing portion being higher. There are government regulations on what constitutes an HDHP with the dollar amounts allowed re-calculated and published each year. In 2021, an HDHP needed to have a deductible of at least $1,400 (if you have an individual plan) or $2,800 for a family plan. The IRS adjusts these values yearly. There are other factors involved in determining if a plan can be considered an HDHP. But the high deductible is a major giveaway. Also, the plan's out-of-pocket maximum must be no higher than $7000 individual and $14,000 family.

For younger and healthier consumers who do not expect to incur many healthcare-related costs, an HDHP may be the right choice because of the lower premium, while it still provides that catastrophic coverage if the unexpected happens. However, for families or those who expect to have higher healthcare-related costs, an HDHP may not be a wise choice.

In addition to lower premiums, an HDHP is usually coupled with a health savings account (HSA) that is meant to fund some of your medical expenses. And in many cases, the HSA is partially funded by the employer. You may also make pre-tax contributions to an HSA and withdrawals are non-taxable as long as they are used for qualifying medical expenses. Health savings accounts are described more fully in a later chapter.

If you want to know more about the differences between PPO plans and HDHPs and the issues that you could have if you select an HDHP, there is a very good article from May 2018 by John C. Goodman, one of the nation's leading thinkers on health policy, and president of the Goodman Institute for Public Policy Research. He published a very comprehensive article in Forbes magazine called "High-Deductible Health Insurance: The Good, the Bad and the Ugly" (Goodman, 2018).

Consider this simple example:

Martha is single, and she is offered health insurance by her employer. Martha chooses the HDHP option that has a deductible of $1750 and a low premium because she is young, is in good shape, and does not expect to incur many medical bills in the next year. The plan is coupled with an HSA, and her employer deposits $500 into her HSA at the beginning of the year. Martha has also decided to make weekly contributions to her HSA using the savings from the lower premiums. She contributes $10 per week before taxes, which equals around $500 for the year. As you know, Martha is responsible for most of her healthcare costs until she reaches her deductible of $1,750. As she begins to incur healthcare costs, she pays for them from her HSA. And Martha pays close attention to her healthcare costs because they are all are being paid from HSA balance. If her healthcare costs for the year are less than $1,000, she has money in her account to cover all the expenses. If something unforeseeable happens and she has high healthcare costs, then after she spends what is in her HSA, now she is only $750 from meeting her deductible where coinsurance begins to apply.

You can also see how this kind of arrangement helps Martha make smarter decisions about her healthcare spending since she wants to keep her costs below $1,000 if possible. But if you are considering this option, make sure you can cover the maximum OOP costs in the event of something catastrophic. The OOP limit in these types of plans is $7,000 (2021) or more. In Martha's case, she would need to be able to afford another $6,000 if she suffered a major illness or accident. The OOP limit on a PPO plan is generally much lower. But since she is young and healthy, she is willing to take this risk. Most HDHP plans also work in conjunction with a PPO network and have the same kind of reduced benefits for out-of-network providers.

Comparing PPO Plans and HDHPs

Let's pause and compare the PPO plan and HDHPs discussed above side by side.

Traditional PPO plan	HDHP

Lower deductible	Higher deductible
Lower out-of-pocket limits	Higher out-of-pocket limits
Higher premium	Lower premium
Not eligible for an HSA	Eligible for an HSA
Employers do not subsidize your deductible	Employers often subsidize your deductible through an HSA

It all depends on your situation. If you are considering a high deductible plan, you should consider all the topics in the table above.

In addition to PPO plans and HDHPs, there are several other types of plans that are less often used. Here are some high-level descriptions of these plan types.

Health Maintenance Organization (HMO) Plans

As the name suggests, HMOs were created to focus on preventative treatments or health maintenance. Like a PPO, an HMO gives you access to certain providers within its network. But unlike PPO plans, services under an HMO plan are covered *only* if you see a provider within the HMO's network. There are no out-of-network benefits. There may be exceptions, but they are usually minimal. They are also typically more restrictive in the coverage they provide, such as allowing only a certain number of visits, tests or treatments.

Most HMOs require you to select a primary care physician (PCP), who will manage your healthcare much like a general contractor manages a construction project. Your PCP will determine what treatments you need and bring in other professionals to assist with your care as needed. Your PCP will refer you to specialists if he or she determines specialized care is necessary. Usually, costs for specialists will not be covered without a PCP referral.

In contrast, PPOs do not require selection of a PCP, and you can see a specialist without a referral in most cases. Since HMO patients need referrals from their PCP to see a specialist, only medically necessary services are approved, and this keeps healthcare and therefore premium costs down. If you choose to see a doctor outside the network, there is no coverage, and you will be responsible for the entire cost of medical services. Premiums are generally lower for HMO plans, and there is usually no deductible or a low one.

Comparing PPOs and HMOs

Traditional PPO plan	HMO plan
More flexibility when picking a doctor or hospital	More restrictive about PCP selection
Involves a network of	Involves a network of
Fewer restrictions on seeing non-network providers. (PPO will pay at a lower rate)	More restrictions on seeing non-network providers. (HMO will not pay at all)
You can see the doctor or specialist you'd like without having to see a PCP first.	Must have a referral to see a specialist
Premiums tend to be higher	Premiums tend to be lower
Usually involves a	Often does not have a
More coverage with fewer restrictions	Less coverage and more restrictions

Point of Service (POS) Plans

A POS plan is a combination of an HMO and a PPO. Typically, POS plans have a network that functions like a PPO. First, you select a primary care physician (PCP), who then manages and coordinates your care within the network. The PCP becomes responsible for making recommendations as far as courses of treatment, specialist visits, medications, and more, like an HMO.

Where a POS plan differs is that it allows you to use a provider who is not in the network. However, like a PPO, if you choose to go out-of-network for your care, you will pay more as a result. In-network providers and specialists are favored.

The term "point of service" is used to show that you make the choice of the provider at the time or "point" of receiving the treatment. These plans are known as point-of-service plans because each time you need healthcare (the time or point of service), you can decide to stay in-network, or you can decide to go outside the network and pay more.

These types of plans only represent a small fraction of health insurance plans. They are usually lower cost but can have a limited number of in-network providers. A referral is still required to see a specialist.

Exclusive Provider Organization (EPO) Plans

An EPO, like a POS, is a hybrid of an HMO and a PPO. Like a PPO, the plan offers a network of doctors and hospitals. But like an HMO, you are responsible for paying out-of-pocket if you seek care from a provider outside your plan's network.

One of the biggest perks of an EPO plan is that you do not need a referral to see a specialist. Premiums for EPOs are usually less than PPOs and overall are often more affordable than PPO plans if you choose a doctor or specialist in your local network. However, if you choose to get care out of your plan's network, your medical care may not be covered.

Minimum Essential Coverage (MEC) Plans

The term "minimal essential coverage" is taken from the Affordable Care Act (ACA), described in a later chapter. This law was passed in 2010, and it says that everyone (with a few exceptions) needs to have a health insurance plan that meets certain minimum standards, and contains what the law defines as minimum essential coverage. MEC plans existed before the Affordable Care Act, and the concept of what is considered Minimal is essentially the same. They have gained popularity in recent years because they can be structured in a way that they satisfy the MEC requirements of the ACA, and allow employers to avoid the Employer Mandate penalties that the ACA imposed, while being affordable because they *only* offer minimal benefits.

MEC plans generally cover preventive and wellness-related tests and treatments only. While they meet the requirements outlined under the ACA, they are not what most think of as traditional health insurance plans. These kinds of plans are often offered by employers with low-wage workers or employers with few employees who want to offer their workers something that the company can afford.

Because MEC plans only offer minimal coverage, the premiums are less than traditional health insurance plans. However, since they offer only the most basic level of required benefits, they are not usually viewed favorably by employees. Sometimes these plans are combined with other minimal benefit plans and together they offer a level of benefits that are more attractive to employees and more affordable than traditional health insurance plans.

Supplemental Insurance Plans

In addition to what traditional health insurance plans cover (medical, dental, vision, etc.), there are several other types of insurance plans available to consumers that deal with very specific illnesses or circumstances. These are often referred to as supplemental or secondary policies as they are additional insurance plans that complement, or are in addition to your primary health insurance.

Critical illness (CI) and long-term care (LTC) insurance are two of the most popular supplemental plans. Critical illness plans provide coverage in the event of illnesses such as cancer, major organ transplants, strokes, heart attacks, and kidney failure. Some plans are specific to one particular illness, while others combine illnesses. When diagnosed according to the rules of the plan, the plan will pay a cash benefit, and often has a minimum daily benefit as well as a policy maximum. Long-term care insurance can help protect your assets, as well as give you better control of your finances, when you need long-term care.

In addition to CI and LTC, other types of policies often seen are accident insurance, hospital insurance, disability insurance, and gap insurance.   Descriptions of each of these types of plans can be found below.

Narrow Network Plans

In a narrow network plan, there is a network of providers; however, there are fewer providers. The premiums are usually lower, and you must use a network provider to receive any benefits. Narrow networks are good for healthier younger people who have less of a need to use a provider. Narrow networks are regulated to ensure that the network contains a mixture of providers in all specialties so that all of a person's healthcare needs can be met by using in-network providers.

Fixed Indemnity Plans

Indemnity plans are a category of health insurance plans called limited benefit plans. They are limited benefit plans because they pay a fixed amount regardless of the charge. It does not matter how high the bills are, these plans will only pay a limited amount. It is called fixed indemnity because it will pay a fixed amount based on the number of occurrences of something. For example, you may have an indemnity plan that pays a benefit of $150 per day in the hospital and $25 per X-ray or diagnostic lab. If you have this plan and you have a three-day hospital stay and on a separate occasion have an X-ray taken, the plan would pay you $150 for each day in the hospital ($450) and $25 for the day you had X-rays taken. That's a benefit of $475 in addition to any other benefit that your regular insurance pays (assuming you also have a traditional health insurance plan), even if the other insurance paid the entire charged amount.

Indemnity insurance plans are often supplemental, meaning they are in addition to a major medical plan. The Obama administration in 2014 tried to make it so indemnity plans could not be sold as stand-alone plans since they do not contain the benefits the ACA requires. However, the courts disagreed, and indemnity plans can in-fact now be sold as stand-alone insurance plans. You should keep in mind that they do not contain the minimum benefits required by the ACA, nor do they contain some of the important protections.

The most well-known provider of indemnity plans is Aflac. Fixed indemnity insurance plans pay a set benefit per specified medical expense, as opposed to a share of the cost. The fixed benefits from these types of plans are paid regardless of other insurance you have. The benefit paid can be used to help pay the deductible, coinsurance, and copays of another health insurance plan, but can also be used to simply offset costs if there is no other insurance plan.

The money received from an indemnity insurance plan can be used to cover whatever expenses you have such as mortgage, rent, and utility payments, child care; and groceries.

Gap Insurance Plans

Gap insurance plans are also limited benefit plans. And, some fixed indemnity plans are structured in a way that allows them to be called gap plans.   They do not pay based on the number of occurrences of things like hospital stays. These plans are intended to help pay the large deductible in some plans. As more and more people are attracted to the low premiums of an HDHP, the number of people enrolled in gap insurance plans is increasing. Remember, along with attractive rates come very high deductible amounts, which could be as high as $7,000 or more.

Gap plans can also include critical illness, accident, or other supplemental types of plans. If that is the case, it might be referred to as a critical illness gap plan, for instance.

Short-Term Insurance Plans

A short-term insurance plan is exactly what it says. It is an insurance plan that is only intended to be in effect for a short amount of time. These plans are useful during times of personal transition, such as being between jobs or you are waiting for a more complete health insurance option to become effective. You can pick your length of coverage, get fast coverage, and drop coverage with no penalty. And the premiums are going to be much less than a marketplace plan or COBRA (described later in this guide). These plans, like gap plans, do not meet the minimum essential coverage requirements of the ACA. Also, you are not guaranteed to get coverage if you have a pre-existing condition. You will have to answer a series of medical questions when you apply.

Prescription Medicine or Rx

A traditional medical plan such as a PPO plan, HMO plan, or HDHP will usually have a prescription drug benefit included. The prescription portion of the plan will probably be administered by a different administrator called a pharmacy benefit manager. The pharmacy or Rx portion of a plan will have its own benefits, and it may even have a separate deductible. The expenses you incur from prescription medicine may or may not get included in the deductible and OOP buckets of your medical plan. It depends on how your plan is structured. You will rarely have a stand-alone pharmacy plan that covers only prescription medicine, but it is possible. Some plans, instead of including a traditional deductible/OOP model for your prescription drugs, will simply offer a discount card that can be used at the pharmacy to obtain prescriptions at a reduced cost.

i

> *The word* prescription *is a compound word containing* pre- *(before) and* script *(written). It refers to the fact that the prescription is an order that must be written down before a drug can be dispensed.* Rx *which is often used as an abbreviation for prescription, comes from the Latin word* recipe *or* recipere *which means "take".*

CHAPTER 4

Health Insurance Bank Accounts

There are three types of accounts most often offered to people as part of their health insurance plan. This chapter explains the types of accounts, and how they are used in combination with your traditional medical health insurance benefits.

The three common accounts are the health savings account (HSA), healthcare reimbursement arrangement (HRA), and the flexible spending account (FSA). While all types of accounts are similar in that the funds can be used to pay for qualified medical expenses before taxes, there are some key differences.

Sometimes employers offer a combination of these accounts to their employees since the accounts operate differently. Also, since tax is not collected on the contributions to these accounts, there are very strict IRS rules about how the money can be used.

Health Savings Account (HSA)

An HSA, as the name says, is a special kind of "savings" account that is used to pay for certain medical expenses. To qualify for an HSA, you have to be enrolled in a high-deductible health plan. An HSA is used to help defray some of the out-of-pocket costs of the high deductible plan. It is frequently partially funded by the employer.

Once an HSA is set up, an employee can contribute additional money to the HSA via a payroll deduction from gross income. Contributions can also be made outside payroll deduction (using money already taxed) and those deposits can be used as deductions on federal tax returns. Interest or earnings on the money in the account is also tax-free. And the employee does not need to pay taxes on withdrawals used to pay for qualified medical expenses. Contributions can be made by the person who owns the account or by an employer (or anyone else who wants to contribute on behalf of the account owner).

A withdrawal from an HSA can be used for a broad range of medical expenses. This includes eyeglasses, contacts, chiropractic care and prescription drugs as well as doctor visits and hospital stays. And the account can also be used to pay for the medical expenses of a spouse or other family members – even if they aren't covered by your HDHP.

One of the advantages of a health savings account is that it is a portable account. The account belongs to the employee. Therefore, the employee can keep the account if they change jobs. Another advantage is that the funds can roll over from year-to-year. So, the account can continue to grow and collect interest until the funds are needed.

<u>Flexible Spending Account (FSA)</u>

A flexible spending account is similar to an HSA, but there are a few key differences that you should be aware of. Similar to an HSA, any money contributed to an FSA is tax-free, and the funds can then be used to pay for certain out-of-pocket healthcare costs. You can use the money in the FSA to pay for things like copayments, deductibles, prescription drugs, and even some over-the-counter items. Contributions can be made to the account via payroll deduction from gross income, which means you don't pay taxes on this money. As with an HSA, you will save the amount of the taxes you will have paid on the contribution.

However, the FSA differs from the HSA in the following ways. The first difference you will notice is that one is a "savings" account and the other is a "spending" account. The FSA does not behave like a savings account. It is owned by the employer, is funded by the employee, does not bear interest, and cannot be withdrawn except to pay for qualified medical expenses. With an FSA, the following rules apply:

- Withdrawals can be made to pay for medical expenses, childcare expenses, and certain commuting expenses.

- You have to declare how much you want your employer to deduct from your gross pay to fund your FSA at the beginning of each calendar year. Once that declaration is made, you generally can't change it until the following year. If you have not elected to have an FSA during the open enrollment period, you probably have to wait until the next open enrollment.

- Your FSA funds must be spent within the tax year. Sometimes a grace period is granted by your employer or you might be allowed to carry over up to $500 but not both. Usually, the money you contribute will be lost if you don't spend it all by the deadline.

The following table compares the two types of accounts.

FSA	HSA
Your employer owns the account	You own the account
The amount you can contribute is set by the IRS but is a different amount for each of the account types.	
You don't have to be covered under a health insurance policy	You must have a high deductible health plan
Interest is not earned on the account	Interest is earned on the account tax free
Unused contributions are lost at the end of the year	Unused contributions roll over to the next year
You and your employer can contribute	
You can only access what has been contributed	You can access entire yearly election
You elect the contribution amount at the beginning of the year	You can change the contribution amount at any time
You lose the account and forfeit funds after a job change	You keep the account after a job change
Funds can be used for childcare and commuting expenses	Funds can be used for qualified medical expenses only

> *The following IRS publications apply to both types of accounts.*
>
> *IRS Publication 502 - list of qualified medical expenses:*
> *https://www.irs.gov/pub/irs-pdf/p502.pdf*
>
> *IRS Publication 969 - information on the tax treatment of HSAs and FSAs:*
> *https://www.irs.gov/publications/p969*

Health Reimbursement Arrangement (HRA)

There are several types of HRAs, but they all offer essentially the same benefit and work the same way. This section describes the general characteristics of an HRA.

A health reimbursement arrangement, sometimes called a health reimbursement account, is an employer-funded, tax-advantaged health benefit used to reimburse employees for out-of-pocket medical expenses and personal health insurance premiums. However, the word "account" is misleading because it is not an actual account, it is an arrangement. An agreement between you and your employer.

The main difference between an HSA and an HRA to you is that the HRA does not allow employee contributions, and while an HSA is combined with a health insurance plan, an HRA is completely separate. Some small employers offer an HRA to their employees, and do not offer health insurance at all.

An HRA can reimburse any expense considered to be a qualified medical expense under IRS section 213(d) of the Internal Revenue Code (also listed in IRS Publication 502), including premiums for personal health insurance policies. This is another difference between an HSA and an HRA because you cannot use HSA funds to pay for premiums.

The employer provides the funds used in an HRA. It is called an account, but it is not an account because reimbursement is made after expenses are incurred. The employer does not need to do any pre-funding. An employee submits proof of expenses incurred to their employer. The employer reviews the employee submitted expenses, and if it is an approved type of expense, the business reimburses the employee with tax-free money.

If an HRA is offered to employees in lieu of an insurance plan, it serves the same purpose as insurance, reimbursing employees for medical expenses up to a particular limit. But the administration of the benefit is completely under the control of the employer.

CHAPTER 5

Medicare

Medicare is a not a type of plan, but a program run by the U.S. federal government. The information in previous chapters about components and types of plans will help you understand the Medicare program better. But Medicare deserves a separate chapter because of its complexity. There are entire books dedicated to the topic of Medicare and there is a wealth of information about Medicare published by the federal government. This chapter will give you an understanding of the components of Medicare, how they are administered, and where to go if you want additional information on the topic of Medicare. (At the end of this chapter, you will find the Medicare website and phone number.)

In the 1960s, the average life expectancy in the United States was sixty-nine to seventy years. People over sixty-five years of age were finding it very difficult to find reasonably priced private health insurance coverage (if they were even accepted), because they were considered a risk because of their advanced age and likelihood of failing health. In 1965, Pres. Lyndon B. Johnson created Medicare and Medicaid to help improve the health and longevity of older Americans. The management of the Medicare program originally fell under the Healthcare Financing Administration (HCFA), which was part of the Department of Health, Education and Welfare. In 1979, the Department of Education was created to stand on its own, and the HEW was renamed to the Department of Health and Human Services (HHS). The HCFA was renamed the Centers for Medicare and Medicaid Services.

HHS was created to protect the health of all Americans and provide essential human services. CMS is the agency within HHS that oversees and administers the nation's major healthcare programs. These include Medicare, Medicaid, the Children's Health Insurance Program, and the state and federal health insurance marketplaces.

Medicare is a federal-government-managed program that provides reduced-cost health insurance if you are sixty-five years of age or older, under sixty-five years of age and receiving social security disability insurance (SSDI) for a certain amount of time, or under sixty-five years of age and with end-stage renal disease (ESRD). Anyone who is entitled to Medicare benefits is considered a "Medicare beneficiary". This chapter deals primarily with Medicare that is available for those sixty-five years of age and older. The program is largely funded by the social security and Medicare taxes you pay on your income and through premiums from Medicare beneficiaries. A portion of the funding comes from the federal government. This is a benefit that you are entitled to as a result of being employed and paying payroll taxes for a certain number of years, similar to your entitlement to social security benefits.

Original Medicare and Medicare Advantage

Medicare has three parts.

- Part A: hospital insurance that covers inpatient care in hospitals, skilled nursing care, hospice and some home healthcare.

- Part B: medical insurance that covers doctors and other providers, lab tests, wellness visits, and outpatient care

- Part D: prescription drug coverage

Parts A and B are referred to as "original Medicare" because when the program was originally established in 1965 it consisted of only those two parts.

Medicare Part D was originally proposed by Pres. Bill Clinton in 1999 and then by Pres. Bush in 2002. The final bill was enacted as part of the Medicare Modernization Act of 2003.

Medicare Part C, is a name given to something called "Medicare Advantage" plans that are bundled plans that cover Parts A, B and usually D and are managed by private insurance companies. These plans often contain additional benefits.

According to data from CMS, as of February 2020, there are over 62 million people enrolled in some type of Medicare plan. Roughly sixty percent of those (37.5 million) are enrolled in original Medicare. Approximately 25 million people are enrolled in Medicare Advantage plans. Over 47 million people are enrolled in some kind of prescription drug plan. (CMS.gov, 2020) CMS estimates that total Medicare spending reached eight hundred billion dollars in 2019 and projected it would reach eight hundred fifty-eight billion in 2020.

Even though Medicare and social security are both programs offered to seniors in the United States based on payroll taxes you paid, it gets a little confusing when you discuss them together because you qualify for the two programs in different ways. Here are some bullet points to help show the complexity of these programs:

- You can begin receiving social security benefits at age sixty-two (or younger if you have a disability)

- You can begin receiving Medicare at age sixty-five.

- You will not receive *full* social security benefits until your full retirement age (FRA). FRA is between sixty-five (if you were born 1937 or before) and sixty-seven years of age (if you were born after 1960).

- If you are receiving social security benefits, then Medicare Part A is free as long as you have worked for a certain number of years and paid payroll taxes during that time.

- If you are sixty-five years of age but have not yet started receiving social security benefits, you can purchase Medicare Parts A and B.

- In most cases, if you buy Part A, you must also buy Part B.

- You can purchase Part B *without* purchasing Part A.

When you turn sixty-five years old, you *must* apply for Medicare. If you are already receiving social security benefits, Part A is free, but you will pay for Part B. If you have not yet started to collect Social Security benefits, then you can still purchase Part A and Part B or just Part B.

Once you are enrolled in Medicare, Parts A and B function in a way very similar to other private or employer sponsored health insurance plans. There are deductibles, copays, and coinsurance. However, there is no yearly limit on out-of-pocket expenses. Since there can still be out-of-pocket expenses after you are enrolled in Medicare, you can purchase supplemental insurance to help cover those expenses. These plans are called gap plans, or Medigap plans.

Original Medicare (Parts A and B) and Part D are administered by the U.S. federal government. Medicare Advantage plans are administered by private insurance companies but still must follow the federal Medicare guidelines. Although all Medicare claims, including Medicare Advantage plan claims, are funded by the federal government, Medicare often sub-contracts some of the administrative functions (such as processing and paying claims) to private companies.

Medicare Advantage plans can have lower out of pocket costs than original Medicare, but in most cases, there is a physician's network involved, so you will have to use providers that are in-network and you may need to have a referral to see a specialist. You will have to ask your provider if they participate in any Medicare Advantage plans to determine if they are in-network. Medicare Advantage plans often also include additional benefits such as vision, hearing and dental coverage.

You will have to pay a premium for a Medicare Advantage plan. Since they usually include more benefits than original Medicare, the premiums are higher. If you are entitled to free Part A coverage and enroll in a Medicare Advantage plan, the Medicare Advantage premium will take that into consideration. Under Medicare Advantage, there are several different plan types just like traditional health insurance plans. You can have an HMO, PPO, POS or several other types of Medicare Advantage plans.

Like a traditional health insurance plan with network affiliation, Medicare providers agree to accept discounts for the services they provide. In this case, they will be part of the Medicare network. The term that is used is Medicare participating.

Just like other networks, Medicare has a list of rates that Medicare providers are obligated to accept called a fee schedule. These rates are called the "Medicare approved amount" or "Medicare allowable". A fee schedule is a complete list of fees used by Medicare to pay doctors or other providers/suppliers. CMS develops fee schedules for physicians, ambulance services, clinical laboratory services, and durable medical equipment, prosthetics, orthotics, and supplies (CMS.gov, 2019). The fees in the fee schedule are adjusted by Medicare based on the geographic location of the provider.

i

> BEWARE: It is possible that a provider may accept Medicare payments, but not accept the Medicare approved amount as payment in full. These providers are considered "non- participating" even though they accept Medicare payments. These providers may advertise "accepting Medicare patients". By law, even if they are non-participating, they cannot charge more than fifteen percent over the Medicare approved amount to anyone enrolled in a Medicare plan.

Even if you continue to work beyond your sixty fifth birthday, or are over sixty-five years of age and covered by a spouse's insurance, you are still entitled to Medicare coverage. If a beneficiary has both Medicare and other health insurance, then Medicare is considered the secondary payer. When Medicare began, if a person was entitled to Medicare (and enrolled), then Medicare paid their claims (with a few exceptions). However, in 1980 Congress passed legislation that made Medicare the secondary payer, if other health insurance exists. The purpose of this law was to protect the trust fund from which Medicare payments are made. The law requires that anyone who bills Medicare for services has the responsibility to determine if Medicare is the primary or secondary payer for those services.

It is not always that straight forward. Medicare becomes the primary payer in certain circumstances if certain conditions are met (for disabled people, people with end-stage-renal-disease, retirees, COBRA, etc.) The complete rules for determining primary and secondary payer status are beyond the scope of this guide.

Medicare Part D

As discussed above, the Part A and Part B Medicare programs are run by the federal government and CMS. Part D plans however are privatized and Medicare contracts with private insurance companies to sell Part D insurance coverage. The Part D program is regulated by

Medicare, and the insurance companies receive subsidies from Medicare to help control costs to the consumers. To have Part D coverage, beneficiaries must purchase a policy offered by one of these companies, which could be a Part D-only plan or a Medicare Advantage plan that includes Part D coverage.

Part D coverage works in a way that is very similar to the way other health insurance plans work. Part D coverage has deductibles, copays and coinsurance. However, CMS explains it differently. According to CMS, your prescription drug plan costs may change during the year depending on the coverage stage you are in, the prescription drugs you use, the pharmacy you use, and other factors. There are four different CMS coverage stages: deductible (if applicable), initial coverage, coverage gap, and catastrophic coverage. Each of the stages is explained below.

Annual Deductible Stage:

This stage begins when you fill your first prescription of a plan year. You pay the full cost of your prescriptions until your spending adds up to the amount of your Part D deductible. If you have no deductible, then you move right on to the next stage. Do not confuse this deductible bucket with the medical deductible bucket discussed previously. This is an entirely separate Medicare Part D deductible bucket.

Initial Coverage Stage:

This stage begins when you meet your plan deductible or immediately if you have no deductible. In this stage, your plan is subject to copayments and coinsurance as described in your plan. There is a limit set by Medicare that determines when this stage ends.

Coverage Gap (Donut Hole) Stage:

This is where it gets a little tricky. This stage begins when you reach the limit of the previous stage specified by CMS. If you do not reach that limit, then you will not reach this stage. Not everyone will enter the coverage gap. This stage has an out-of-pocket limit (for drugs only) that is set by CMS. In 2020, it is $6,350. Your Part D OOP bucket will contain your deductible amount, what you paid in copays and coinsurance in the previous stage, and what you pay for medications while you are in the coverage gap. This is a special Part D only OOP bucket.

In this stage, the plan is temporarily limited in how much it pays for your prescription medicine. For example, in 2020, Part D coverage paid for five percent of the cost of covered brand-name drugs, and the drug manufacturer gave a seventy percent discount. The amount you paid was twenty-five percent. The good news is (and it really is good news) that the amount you pay (twenty-five percent) and the seventy percent discount you got from the manufacturer both count as out-of-pocket spending and go into the Medicare Part D OOP bucket. Medicare also pays for seventy-five percent of the price for generic drugs when you're in the coverage gap.

Catastrophic Coverage Stage:

This stage begins when you exit the previous stage (coverage gap) because your Medicare Part D out-of-pocket spending reached the limits set by CMS for that year. In the catastrophic stage, you will pay a low coinsurance or copayment amount, set by CMS, for all of your covered prescription drugs. That means the plan and the government pay for the rest – about ninety-five percent of the cost. You will remain in this phase until the end of the plan year.

Medicare Fraud

The Medicare program is fraught with fraud. It is likely that some providers (as well as other opportunists) think it is easy to commit fraud because it's a federal government-run program full of red-tape. They probably think it should be easy to defraud Medicare because with all that red tape it would take forever to realize someone was abusing the system. Both are true. It is easy to defraud the Medicare system if that's what you want to do. And it might take a while to catch you. But, a great deal of effort is put into finding and prosecuting Medicare abusers. If you read the chapter on fraud, you will see some great examples of people who have been caught committing Medicare fraud.

According to a Government Accountability Office (GAO) report from March 2019, "Medicare faces a significant risk with improper payments—payments that either were made in an incorrect amount or should not have been made at all—which reached an estimated $48 billion in fiscal year 2018". (GAO.gov, 2019). Part of the Affordable Care Act involves reducing Medicare Fraud to reduce the overall cost of the program. According to a 2016 article on the website theFiscalTimes.com, the Obama administration reported to Congress that it had "prevented $42 billion of improper payments to doctors and other medical providers in fiscal years 2013 and 2014" and from 2010 through 2016 "the administration's fraud taskforce arrested and prosecuted about 1,200 people allegedly involved in defrauding Medicare and Medicaid of more than $3.5 billion dollars" (Pianin, 2016).

CMS encourages anyone who suspects Medicare fraud to report it by calling 1-800-HHS-TIPS. They also give you the ability to report suspected fraud online, by FAX, or by email. According to CMS you can remain anonymous; however, they offer rewards to whistleblowers if fraud is found, convictions are obtained, and money is recovered.

Medicaid & CHIP

Medicaid and CHIP are joint federal and state programs operated by the states within the federal Medicare guidelines, for people with low incomes, children, and pregnant women. Although the federal government pays a portion of the costs, Medicaid is administered and operated by the states, and each state's program is a little different depending on the needs and goals of that state. Each state runs different Medicaid-funded programs, and it is even possible that the Medicaid program in your state goes by some other name.

Each state uses its own financial eligibility guidelines to determine whether you are eligible for Medicaid coverage. If you are eligible for Medicare and Medicaid (dually eligible), you can enroll in both. Medicaid can cover services that Medicare does not, such as Medicare's out-of-pocket costs (deductibles, coinsurances, copayments).

For information about Medicaid, you can go to the Medicaid website www.medicaid.org. Every state has a different contact for questions about Medicaid. You can determine the Medicaid contact for your state, or you can contact the Centers for Medicare and Medicaid Services at 877-267-2323. You can also send an email to the Medicaid.gov mailbox: Medicaid.gov@cms.hhs.gov

CHIP stands for the Children's Health Insurance Program which provides low-cost health coverage to children in families that earn too much money to qualify for Medicaid. As with Medicaid, CHIP operates differently in every state, including the rules for who qualifies. CHIP works closely with Medicaid. If you apply for Medicaid coverage, you'll also find out if your children qualify for CHIP. If they qualify, you won't have to buy an insurance plan to cover them.

According to Medicaid.gov, there were 70,609,251 people enrolled in Medicaid and CHIP in the 51 states that reported enrollment data for December 2019. Additionally, 35,085,794 individuals were enrolled in CHIP or were children enrolled in the Medicaid program in the 49 states that reported child enrollment data for December 2019. (Medicaid.gov, 2019)

Summary

One of the major components of the Affordable Care Act deals with Medicare. The goals were to reduce cost and make the program more efficient. It increased the number of people eligible for subsidies by raising the income levels for receiving subsidies (referred to as expanding Medicare), and it also contained several activities aimed at reducing fraud. So, in the end, the plan was to make sure those who are on Medicare are deserving of Medicare benefits, and make Medicare more affordable and available to more people.

People have been paying payroll taxes into the Medicare trust since Medicare was created in 1965, but the health of the Medicare trust is in question. Some experts warn that the Medicare trust will be insolvent by the year 2026. But Medicare actually consists of several different trusts and is not in danger of insolvency any time soon. The level of federal government funding for Medicare is a topic of conversation with every federal budget proposal.

To obtain more information about Medicare, you can go to the Medicare website at www.medicare.gov, or call 1-800-MEDICARE (1-800-633-4227).

*Information in this chapter was obtained from federal government publications "The Official U.S. Government Medicare Handbook" (CMS.gov, 2020) and "Your Guide to Medicare Prescription Drug Coverage" (CMS.gov, 2020)

CHAPTER 6

Signing Up / Enrollment

This chapter focuses on how to obtain health insurance and some of the rules that have been established for applying. As you will see, there may be different ways to apply, and different rules about when and how you apply depending on what kind of insurance plan you are trying to obtain.

Open Enrollment

The process of signing up for health insurance is usually referred to as "enrolling" during a certain period called an "enrollment period". You have surely heard the term open enrollment. This is a generic term that refers to the period during which you can select coverage, change your existing coverage, or drop coverage under a health insurance plan. Basically, the plan is "open" for enrollment during this period. Unless you are purchasing private health insurance from an insurance company, you will experience an Open Enrollment period. Open Enrollment periods usually occur once per year and are usually held in the last few months of the calendar year. Most plan years run January to December, but that is not always the case. The reason that open enrollment periods exist is to keep you from only obtaining health insurance only when you are sick.

If you do not enroll in a health insurance plan, or change your coverage during the open enrollment period, you usually must wait an entire year, until the next open enrollment period to make the change. However, there is something called a qualifying event that sometimes allows an exception to be made. A qualifying event is a life change that significantly alters your need for health insurance or level of coverage. If a qualifying event, or qualifying life event occurs, you are generally given a specific number of days to make a change in your coverage regardless of the time of year. Typical qualifying life events include but are not limited to the following:

- The birth or adoption of a child
- Marriage and divorce
- Loss of other coverage
- Becoming a U.S. citizen

You will also read about qualifying events in the section on COBRA later in this guide. The COBRA qualifying event is similar but only applies to events that cause loss of coverage and allow a person to become eligible for COBRA coverage.

Employer-Sponsored and Private Health Insurance Plans

Open enrollment periods apply to employer-sponsored health insurance plans as well as private health insurance plans, including those purchased on the HealthCare.gov marketplace or one of the state exchanges.

For employer-sponsored plans, your company's human resources department will usually coordinate the open enrollment period and let you know how to enroll.

For plans purchased on the marketplace, you can enroll online at HealthCare.gov, or by telephone at 1-800-318-2596; you can contact an agent, broker or enrollment assister; or you can complete a paper application and mail it to them.

There are also numerous companies who sell private health insurance plans online or through agents and brokers. You do not need to wait for an open enrollment period if you purchase one of these plans outside HealthCare.gov.   Although these plans may comply with ACA requirements, you should be prepared to pay a higher premium, and you will not be eligible for any of the subsidies (payment assistance) available through HealthCare.gov.

Medicare

There are strict rules about when you sign up for Medicare, and you may need to pay more for your coverage if you do not abide by the rules. If you are under sixty-five years of age but already receiving social security benefits, you will automatically be enrolled in Medicare Parts A and B. Otherwise, you *must* sign up for Medicare three months before you turn sixty-five. If you do not sign up at this time, there could be delays in receiving benefits, and you may have to pay a penalty and higher rates for as long as you have Part B coverage.

If you are covered by an employer-sponsored group health plan when you turn sixty-five because you either still working or covered by a spouse's policy, then you do not need to sign up for Medicare. If this is the case, then you can sign up for Part A and Part B during a "special enrollment period". This just means that you can sign up without penalty at any time you remain covered by the group policy or within eight months of losing that coverage. If you have not enrolled during your initial enrollment period, and you do not qualify for a special enrollment period, you can still sign up between January 1 and March 31 each year, but you may be subject to the late enrollment penalty.

Medicaid and CHIP

You can apply for Medicaid at any time during the year; Medicaid and CHIP do not have specific open enrollment periods. And there are two ways that you can apply for Medicaid: (1) through the health insurance marketplace or (2) through your state Medicaid agency.

Fill out a health insurance application through the health insurance marketplace at HealthCare.gov. If it looks like anyone in your household qualifies for Medicaid or CHIP, your information will automatically be sent to your state agency. They will then contact you about enrollment. When you submit your marketplace application, you'll also find out if you qualify for any subsidies. If you qualify for Medicaid coverage, your state agency will also let you know if your children qualify for CHIP.

CHAPTER 7

Low Income Subsidies

Both the federal and state governments provide help paying for health insurance plan premiums for individuals and families who meet certain minimum income standards. This premium assistance is called a "subsidy", and there are many programs that provide subsidies. This chapter provides an overview of different kinds of subsidies available, how you qualify to receive them, and how you apply for them.

Marketplace Subsidies

In a previous chapter you learned that the federal government (and some states' governments) operates a service that helps people shop for and enroll in affordable health insurance plans called the "marketplace" or "exchange". The health insurance marketplace gives consumers the ability to shop for health insurance plans through HealthCare.gov. Some subsidies are available and obtained when purchasing insurance on the marketplace.

Government subsidies are complex in how they are calculated and how they are used. They are also part of many current lawsuits and legislation (proposed and passed) that limit or eliminate certain subsidies. This section provides an overview of subsidies. If you want additional information on marketplace subsidies, you should visit www.healthcare.org. Subsidies are available whether obtaining health insurance on the federal marketplace or one of the state exchanges.

If you plan to purchase your health insurance on the federal marketplace or one of the state exchanges, you may be eligible for one of two types of assistance available. When you go through the application process, you will be asked questions about your income and the number of people in your family/household. The website will perform the calculations and let you know if you qualify for either or both of the subsidies.

The first of these subsidies is called the premium tax credit (PTC). To qualify for the PTC, you need to have income that falls within a certain range, not be a dependent on someone else's return, have insurance purchased on the marketplace, be unable to obtain affordable coverage through an employer, and not be eligible for health insurance through another government program. The income range is one hundred to four hundred percent of the federal poverty level (FPL). According to the federal register, the FPL for a single person, in the forty-eight contiguous states, in 2019 was $12,760 (HHS.gov, 2020). If you make more than four hundred percent of the FPL or less than one hundred percent of the FPL, you will not qualify for marketplace subsidies, but may still qualify for other government assistance. The subsidies are on a sliding scale if your income is between one hundred and four hundred percent of the FPL.

The PTC is a tax credit you receive when filing your federal income taxes, or if eligible, you can have "advance payments" sent directly to your insurance company to reduce your premiums. You can use all, some, or none of your premium tax credit in advance to lower your monthly premium. Since the PTC is based on your income, the estimated PTC that determines your advance payments may be different from your final PTC calculated at the end of the year when your income for the year is known. If you use more advance payments of the tax credit than you qualify for based on your final yearly income, you must repay the difference when you file your federal income tax return. If you use less premium tax credit than you qualify for, you'll get the difference as a refundable credit when you file your taxes. (CMS.gov, 2020)

The second kind of subsidy is the cost-sharing subsidy that is intended to reduce your out-of-pocket healthcare expenses by helping pay copayments, deductibles, and coinsurance. Unlike the PTC, this subsidy is only available to people who enroll in a certain kind of plan (Silver), and the upper-income limit is 250 percent of the FPL.

> *The Trump administration eliminated funding for the cost-sharing subsidies. However, the ACA still requires insurers to provide the subsidies. This just meant that the federal government would no longer reimburse the insurance companies when they extend subsidies to policy holders. In response, the insurance companies were forced to increase their premiums to offset the money they would have received from the government.*

> *Because of 2021 legislation, nearly everyone with an ACA health plan qualified for increased financial help with premiums. Many Americans who bought their own insurance outside the ACA marketplaces qualified for marketplace subsidies after the new law.*
>
> *It is estimated that more than six million people, or about three in five uninsured Americans had the ability to find health plans on Healthcare.Gov with no premiums after the*

Change in Circumstances

If you are receiving marketplace subsidies it is important to report life changes to the marketplace as soon as possible when they occur. Any life change to a parameter used to calculate how much subsidy you qualify for (income, household size, etc.) could potentially decrease or increase the amount of your subsidy. If you qualify for a larger subsidy, you want to get it changed as soon as possible. And if it results in a lower advance PTC subsidy, you should contact the marketplace as soon as possible to avoid owing taxes at the end of the year.

Medicare Subsidies

If you are a Medicare beneficiary or becoming one, there are subsidies and assistance programs available for you as well to assist with Medicare premiums and other medical costs.

You can get help from your state paying your Medicare premiums and other healthcare costs (depending on your income) by programs called Medicare savings programs. These are programs run by the states under the federal guidelines of the Medicare program. There are four kinds of Medicare savings programs:

- Qualified Medicare Beneficiary (QMB) program – this helps pay for Part A and Part B premiums and other costs.
- Specified Low-Income Medicare Beneficiary (SLMB) program – a state program that helps pay for Part B premiums only.
- Qualifying Individual (QI) program – a state program that helps pay for Part B premiums only.
- Qualified Disabled and Working Individuals (QDWI) program – this helps pay Part A premiums only.

If you qualify for a QMB, SLMB, or QI program, you also automatically qualify to get extra help paying for Medicare prescription drug coverage, which helps seniors with low incomes pay nothing or nearly nothing for prescription medicine. Even if you don't qualify for one of the programs above, and you have limited income, you may qualify for help with the costs of prescription drugs through the program called the Part D low-income subsidy (LIS).

For more information on any of these programs and to see if you qualify, please contact Centers for Medicare and Medicaid Studies (CMS).

Source: (medicare.gov, 2020)

Part III – Now You've Got a Plan

CHAPTER 8

Documents and Other Information

Now that you are enrolled in a health insurance plan, where do you go to get information to learn about the details of your coverage? There are a variety of ways to obtain information about your plan. There are several documents available to you that describe all your benefits and the rights and responsibilities of you and the insurer.

As stated previously, health insurance is complex. And when you add in all the legal wording, you've got dozens or possibly hundreds of pages of information, which few people actually sit down and read. This is unfortunate because there is important information in the documents if you know where to look. Most employers or insurance companies simply make the documents available and expect you to figure out what's important. Often, the full document is loaded onto a website or customer portal, which qualifies as being delivered to you since you now have access to the document(s).

This chapter explains some of the important documents and highlights some of the differences so you are more familiar with the documents you've received for your health insurance and can more easily determine what is important. If you have not already reviewed your health insurance plan's documents, it is important to do so before you need to use your coverage.

Medical ID Card

When you enroll in a health insurance plan, you will receive an ID card. Although this is not a document per se, it is one of the most important items you will possess that contains information about your health insurance coverage. Your health insurance ID card will contain important information about your medical insurance and may include information about other coverage you have such as dental, vision and pharmacy coverage. This card not only informs providers that you actually have health insurance but also contains important information telling a provider what kind of plan you have, who to call if they have questions, where to send claims, and how you should be charged.

The medical ID card is usually about the size of a credit card, so it can be carried in your wallet or purse, and you should carry it with you at all times like you carry your driver's license. You will show this card to every provider you see for medical care. Many insurers and administrators make your insurance ID card available on their portal or the insurer or administrator's website or mobile app.

Plan Documents

Plan documents are different depending on whether the plan is fully-insured or self-insured (Self and Fully Insured are explored later in this guide). Under a fully-insured arrangement, an insurance company (like Blue Cross, Cigna, and Aetna) assumes all the responsibility for paying your claims *and* most of the risk that goes along with it. Just like auto insurance, or homeowner's insurance, they collect premiums from those they insure, pay claims within the rules of the plan, and count on a portion of the insured population having no or a small number of claims to offset those who do. The money to pay claims comes completely from premiums people pay for the insurance.

In a self-insured arrangement, an employer sponsors a health insurance plan for their employees and assumes most of the risk. The employer (the insurer in this case) collects a premium from the insured (their employees) usually through payroll deduction, and they are responsible for paying all claims. For this reason, these types of insurance plans are also referred to as self-funded. A third-party administrator is almost always involved to handle all the administrative tasks associated with paying claims, as well as providing other healthcare-related services. These arrangements are discussed in more detail in a later chapter.

Summary of Benefits and Coverage (SBC)

The SBC is a document that the government says must be provided to all insured people. Not only is the document itself mandated, but the format of the document *must* also follow government guidelines. It is mandated that everyone has access to a copy of this document regarding their health insurance plan. There is important information in this document, but it is not in a very user-friendly format. The document does spell out the plan's deductible and OOP limits, as well as the benefits that you will receive for many often-used medical services.

Important Questions	Answers	Why This Matters:
What is the overall deductible?	For network providers $650 individual / $1,250 family; for out-of-network providers $1,225 individual / $2,425 family	Generally, you must pay all of the costs from providers up to the deductible amount before this plan begins to pay. If you have other family members on the plan, each family member must meet their own individual deductible until the total amount of deductible expenses paid by all family members meets the overall family deductible.
Are there services covered before you meet your deductible?	Yes. Preventive care and second surgical opinions are covered before you meet your deductible.	This plan covers some items and services even if you haven't yet met the deductible amount. But a copayment or coinsurance may apply. For example, this plan covers certain preventive services without cost-sharing and before you meet your deductible. See a list of covered preventive services at https://www.healthcare.gov/coverage/preventive-care-benefits/.
Are there other deductibles for specific services?	Yes. $100 individual / $300 family under prescription drugs	You must pay all of the costs for these services up to the specific deductible amount before this plan begins to pay for these services.
What is the out-of-pocket limit for this plan?	For network providers $1,000 individual / $2,000 family; for out-of-network providers $25,000 individual / $50,000 family	The out-of-pocket limit is the most you could pay in a year for covered services. If you have other family members in this plan, they have to meet their own out-of-pocket limits until the overall family out-of-pocket limit has been met. *The prescription drug section has a separate $2,000 single out-of-pocket limit.*
What is not included in the out-of-pocket limit?	Premiums, deductibles, co-pays, penalties, balance-billing charges, and health care this plan doesn't cover.	Even though you pay these expenses, they don't count toward the out-of-pocket limit

The figure above is one section of a five-page SBC document. This SBC is from the same plan that was used for the examples in earlier chapters. The underlined words are hyperlinks to definitions on HealthCare.gov.

Schedule of Benefits or Summary of Benefits (SOB)

The SOB contains the same information as the SBC but is formatted differently to make the document more readable. Most healthcare and health insurance professionals as well as many consumers agree that it is easier to understand than an SBC. A sample of the SOB for the same plan we have been using is shown next.

	In-Network	Non-Network
Calendar Year Deductible:		
Per Covered Person	$ 650	$1,225
Per Family	$1,250	$2,425
Benefit Percentage:		
Health Care Plan Pays	80% of the first $5,000 then 100% thereafter	50% of the first $50,000 then 100% thereafter
Covered Person Pays	20% of the first $5,000	50% of the first $50,000
Out-of-Pocket Maximum:		
Per Covered Person	$1,000	$25,000
Per Family	$2,000	$50,000
The charges for the following do not accrue to the Out-of-Pocket Maximum and are never reimbursed at 100% by the Plan.		

- Deductible
- Co-pays
- Cost Containment Penalties
- Non covered services

- Charges in excess of Usual, Customary and Reasonable or the Allowable Claim Limit
- Prescription Plan has a separate OOP maximum that needs to be met. See Prescription Drug Expense Benefit Section for additional details

Summary Plan Description (SPD)

The federal government requires self-insured employee benefit plans to have a plan document. The plan document is a comprehensive document containing the rights of the participants (both you and your insurer), and guidelines for decisions the administrator needs to make. It also contains a description of the plan's benefits and how the claims are funded. If a plan document exists, then it is accompanied by a document called an SPD, which is another document that is a summary-level description of benefits, just in a different format.

In many cases, the plan document and SPD are in a single document. If this is the case, the document must comply with the federal government's plan document requirements as well as the SPD format and content rules. Some courts have expressed the view that having a combined document is not acceptable because a document cannot summarize itself. However, there are at least two appellate courts that have approved the combined document approach, and that is the way most TPAs operate. The rest of this guide assumes that any reference to an SPD is referencing a combined document.

Although the SPD is a lengthy document, its purpose is to provide plan information to the insured in an understandable form. The SPD is required to contain certain items such as eligibility requirements, claims procedures and circumstances that will lead to loss of benefits.

Although it is called a "summary" document, it contains very detailed benefits information and definitions. It should be a very useful resource if you have a question about whether a specific medical condition or procedure is covered. It is usually very clear about what is *not* covered in a section called "Exclusions". As with the SBC, this document must be made available to all participants in a health insurance plan. Because of its size, it is rarely distributed to participants in hard-copy form. Instead, it is often posted to a company's intranet for participants in the health insurance plan to have as a reference.

Policy

The term policy is usually used with a fully-insured plan, and it can be thought of as a contract that explains the terms and conditions of the health insurance plan. You have surely heard the term insurance policy associated with life, auto, or homeowner's insurance. These are all fully-insured forms of insurance.

If you receive your health insurance from your employer and it is a fully-insured health insurance plan, a policy has most likely been issued to your employer. Your employer has entered into a contract with the insurer, and the insurer collects a premium from your employer. Usually, the employer then collects individual premiums from the employees through payroll deductions. They can collect enough from employees to pay their premium, or they can determine how much they want the employees to contribute, and then supplement the remainder themselves as an employee benefit. If you purchase an individual policy from an insurance company, then the policy will be issued to you, and you alone are responsible for paying the premium to the insurance company.

A policy is sometimes issued to an association, which is a group, comprising individuals (or organizations) with common interests. An association can take advantage of its size to obtain better rates on benefits for the members (not only health insurance). Examples are trade unions, and other professional associations such as the National Education Association (NEA), National Rifle Association (NRA), and American Medical Association (AMA). In the case of an association, a policy is issued to the association.

Certificate

A fully insured plan will have a certificate that is issued to the person insured. If the policy is issued to the employer, then the certificate is issued to the employee. This document will contain information similar to what is in an SPD and describes all of the detailed benefits and provisions of the plan in an understandable form.

The certificate is often referred to as a certificate of insurance (COI) and can be used as proof of insurance. At times, in addition to the certificate, an insurer can provide a one-page summary of benefits to be used as proof of insurance benefits. It's not part of the policy, and it doesn't change the terms of the policy.

Rider

In general, a rider is something that is being added to an insurance policy. The provisions in the rider cannot stand alone. In other words, the rider becomes part of the policy it is attached to. It could be adding an entirely new benefit, or it could be amending the terms of the policy. For instance, there could be a life insurance rider attached to a standard health insurance plan, or a critical illness rider, a dental rider, or almost any other benefit that is added to the original policy. A rider is not needed for a self-insured plan. Because of the flexibility that a self-insured plan has, and the fact that the employer is assuming most of the financial risk, they can add any benefit they want into the at any time, if it is something they want to provide to their employees.

Customer Portal

Most insurers and administrators have a customer portal that allows you to obtain information about your health insurance plan and to communicate with the insurer. The portal is very valuable because it provides not only all the health insurance plan details but also information about how you are using your plan and the status of claims, which you will learn about in Part III. The portal usually also gives you access to your health insurance ID card, which is handy if you are at a provider's office and you do not have your physical ID card with you or if you haven't received your card yet. Some insurers and administrators also have an app version of their portal available for your phone. Most PBMs also have a portal where you can see information about your prescription medicine claims and get information about your plan, and some PBMs allow you to fill mail-order prescriptions right on their portal.

If your insurer doesn't have a portal where you can sign in and receive personalized information about your plan, they will sometimes have a website where you can obtain information about your plan if a common plan is offered to many people. Medicare has a portal for Medicare beneficiaries at https://www.mymedicare.gov. And since as you learned previously Medicaid is run by individual states, the states may have their own portal for their Medicaid participants.

CHAPTER 9

What Happens When
You are Sick or Injured?

Now it's time to actually use the insurance you have selected and are paying a premium for. This chapter describes how your health insurance plan works for you behind the scenes. Most of this occurs without you being aware. But if you understand what is occurring it will help you make better decisions about your healthcare and health insurance, and could save you money.

Provider Networks

You learned in a previous chapter that a provider network is a group of doctors or hospitals and other types of providers who have signed contracts with a network to accept negotiated (discounted) rates for their services. Knowing how your plan works, can help you avoid unexpected medical bills. Certain choices you make can affect what you'll pay out-of-pocket. Knowing the difference between in-network and out-of-network providers will help you save on your healthcare expenses. If a provider or facility has no contract with your health plan's network, they're considered "out-of-network" and can charge you the full price. It's usually much higher than the in-network discounted rate.

When you go to a provider for a service, you often ask, "Do you accept my insurance?" What you are really asking is, "Do you have a contract with my health plan's provider network?" Providers don't really care who pays them as long as they get paid. In essence, providers will accept anyone's money, whether it is coming from insurance or out of your pocket. If they are in your provider network, and insurance is paying, they know that they stand a much better chance of being paid.

After the administrator processes a claim and notifies you and your provider what portion (if any) they are paying, the remainder gets billed to you. That is called balance billing because they are billing you the balance of the charges after the insurance pays. Unfortunately, if you have a serious accident, a major illness, or surgery, you are often seen by dozens of different doctors. Some of them may be out-of-network doctors and you don't even have the opportunity to ask them. In the case of an emergency, you may not have the ability (or desire) to ask. Most health plans make exceptions in emergency situations.

But what if it's a scheduled surgery? You may still get a bill from doctors who treated you at the hospital but are not part of your plan's network. Out-of-network providers often include radiologists, anesthesiologists, pathologists and surgeons helping your in-network surgeon. Your plan may not cover any out-of-network care, leaving you unexpectedly responsible for the entire cost. Or they may cover part of the cost, but at a much lower rate than if the provider was in-network. You may have to pay the difference.

This can be avoided by doing a little up-front work. Tell your doctor in advance that you only want to use in-network providers. If your doctor has specific providers in mind, check with your insurer to make sure they are in your network.

> *Sometimes, a provider you have been seeing for a long time leaves the network they were a part of. The office may not inform you of this change, and the provider may now be out-of-network. Always ask the office staff if the provider is still a member of your network.*

Ask your insurer what you can do to avoid being balance billed. Ask the hospital to help you ensure that any doctors assigned to your case are in your plan's network.

> *Beware: If your insurance changes, your network may change as well. If this occurs, you should receive a new ID card even if you do not change employers. A new network is often introduced for cost savings, and you may need to shop for a different primary care provider. If you receive a new ID card in the mail, make sure you read it to see what has changed from your previous card.*

In-Network versus Out-of-Network Expenses

If you see an out-of-network provider or use a facility that is out of network, then you are probably paying full (not discounted) price. When health insurers don't have a contracted relationship with out-of-network doctors and facilities, they can't control what is charged for services. And rates may be higher than the discounted in-network rate.

If your doctor's bill is higher than what your plan will pay, you might have to pay the difference. Health insurance plans have set amounts that represent the most they'll pay for every possible service received out-of-network. If the doctor or facility charges more than your plan is willing to pay, you could be responsible for paying the difference in addition to your deductible, copay, or coinsurance. In-network doctors and facilities have agreed to accept reimbursement at the network rate and not balance bill for charges above the agreed upon fee.

When you see a provider, a specialist, or use a testing facility of some kind, the office personnel will ask for your health insurance ID card. They will use this card to determine what benefits your health insurance provides. Sometimes, the provider's office can determine your benefits simply by looking at your ID card.   Other times, they may need to contact the insurer.

Some plans require you to pay a small copay to the provider's office at the time of service. Typically, this is in the range of ten to thirty dollars. Sometimes, the provider's office will not require you to pay anything at the time of service. If it is determined that you do not have adequate health insurance coverage, you may be asked to pay the entire charge before you are seen by the provider.

Regardless of how much you pay at the provider's facility, if you have insurance coverage and you receive a billable service of some kind, the provider's office creates a claim that is sent to the insurance company or some other administrator that specializes in processing medical claims. The provider usually sends the claim to the place stated on your ID card.

> *The claim may go somewhere other than the administrator first. If you have seen an in-network provider, the claim may go to someone who will apply the in-network discount before the administrator receives the claim. Or the administrator may perform this function themselves. This is called "repricing"*

The claim will contain (in addition to your identity) specific codes to state the service(s) provided (the *what*), where they were provided (the *where*), how many of the services were provided (the *quantity*), and codes to indicate the "diagnosis" (the *why*).

> *Keep in mind that any medical service could result in more than one claim. There are often providers in the background, performing services as part of your treatment that you never see, such as labs.*

For example, patient Bob has a follow-up appointment at his family doctor to make sure his emphysema (a chronic condition) is being controlled. He also has some blood drawn which is sent to a lab for analysis. In this case, Bob's family doctor is the provider, and the "service" he has received might be one office visit.   The diagnosis is emphysema. The provider's office will create a claim that contains all the information above (represented by a series of codes), including the charges, and send the claim to the health insurance plan's administrator. The medical ID card tells the provider's office where to send the claim. In the above example, the lab-work would result in a separate bill and the lab would create a claim as well. Complex procedures like surgery or other hospital stays could result in multiple claims, submitted by multiple providers.

Claim Processing

Claim processing refers to the process of receiving a claim, reviewing the contents of the claim to identify errors, determining the amount of money to pay the provider or providers, making the actual payment to the provider or providers and making notification to the insured and the provider to explain how the claim was processed. Computer systems are often used to perform claim processing. In addition, insurance companies and administrators have claim processors or analysts to handle more complex claims. Since claims often contain a complex set of codes to describe the service(s) provided as well as your diagnosis, errors can be made regardless of whether a human being or a computer is doing the claim processing.

Once the insurer or administrator receives the claim, they compare it to the type of benefits in the insured's health insurance plan. The possible outcomes after a claim is processed are as follows:

- The claim is *denied*, in which case you will owe the provider whatever was not collected at the time of service. This could be because your health insurance is not in good standing, or the particular service is not covered by your plan, or the claim could have simply been sent to the wrong place. The insurer or administrator will notify you and the provider's office that the claim has been denied, and the provider's office will send you a bill.

- The service is covered. The insurer administrator will most likely send the provider the amount that has not been collected at the time of service minus any deductible or coinsurance obligation you have. The provider will bill you for any remaining balance. This is called "balance billing".

- The insurer or administrator may need more information from you, the provider, or some other party. In this case they request the missing information and hold the claim until the information is received.

For providers who are in-network, you have learned that the network has established and the provider agreed to accept a discounted rate that the network has created. But what about out-of-network providers? Can they charge as much as they want? They pretty much can. But when the insurer determines what they consider to be the allowable charge, they often use something called usual, customary and reasonable (UCR) as a basis and try to force the provider to accept a lower more reasonable reimbursement. HealthCare.gov defines UCR as, "the amount paid for a medical service in a geographic area based on what providers in the area usually charge for the same or similar medical service". Regardless of what the provider charges, the insurance company may only allow up to some percentage of UCR. This is called the "allowable", and the insurer will apply the proper benefit to the allowable and not the full charge.

Insurance administrators scrutinize every claim to look for errors. Other than codes that are incorrect, there are other checks that can be performed to make sure the claim does not contain erroneous charges. For example:

- a hysterectomy for a male patient or vasectomy for a female patient,

- duplicate charges (such as multiple office visits in the same day, or multiple surgeries in the same day),

- three knee replacements,

- a completely duplicate claim,

- an office visit *and* some service that cannot be performed at a doctor's office like inpatient surgery,

- patient cannot be found or is found but has had coverage ended, or the service was performed before the patient's coverage began.

Some of the checks are looking for honest mistakes. There are thousands of possible codes and combinations thereof that a claim could contain, which makes mistakes likely. According to a CNBC news study, "While the American Medical Association estimated that 7.1 percent of paid claims in 2013 contained an error, a 2014 NerdWallet study found mistakes in forty-nine percent of Medicare claims. Groups that review bills on patients' behalf, including Medical Billing Advocates of America and CoPatient, put the error rate closer to seventy or eighty percent" (Grant, 2016) .

Unfortunately, if a provider makes a mistake on your claim, you may not be aware. If you are notified that your claim is denied, it can cause concern and anxiety because you immediately assume you will be responsible for the charges. Be patient and investigate. It is often due to someone's mistake, and clerical or coding errors can be corrected. Often, billing errors go unnoticed and the claim is paid.

Other checks are performed to help recognize fraud. There are literally hundreds of checks that can be performed, and hundreds of ways that can be used to commit fraud on the insurance companies. And fraudsters come up with new methods every day.

If the claim satisfies all the checks, the payment is determined. Depending on the benefits in the plan, how full the deductible bucket and OOP buckets are, the amount of coinsurance, and so on (see examples later in this chapter), a payment will be made. Normally, the payment is made to the provider; but in some cases, the payment is made to you, in which case you may be expected to make payment to the provider yourself. The administrator sends you something called an "Explanation of Benefits (EOB)". The EOB explains how the claim has been processed and what the dollar charges are; and if a network is involved, it will show the discount received on the service(s), the allowable amount(s), and the amount that the insurer actually paid the provider. An "explanation of payment (EOP)" is sent to the provider along with a payment. An EOP is similar to an EOB and allows the provider to link the payment they receive to your balance, explains how the payment has been calculated; or if there is no payment, it explains why.

> *Insurance companies and administrators are required by law to send you an explanation of benefits when your claim is processed. The EOB explains how the insurance company or administrator has processed the claim, and how much of the charge the plan will cover. The administrator sends the provider an explanation of payment which describes why they are receiving a payment or why they are receiving no payment from the insurer for a service they have performed.*

Subrogation

We will not dive too deeply into the topic of subrogation; however, you should be familiar with the term and its meaning.

Subrogation is the process a health insurance company or administrator uses to ensure that the proper party is paying for a health insurance claim. In other words, they make sure they do not pay a claim if in fact, there is someone else who should be responsible for paying it.

Often, when an injury or illness occurs, liability for the payment of claims is with someone other than your health insurance insurer. Usually, the administrator will pay the claims and then do an investigation, or have another company trained in subrogation investigation do the latter. If it is found that a third party is responsible, they will seek reimbursement either from the third party or from you if you have already been reimbursed by the third party. The most typical examples of third-party insurance are automobile insurance, workers' compensation insurance, or scenarios where a court has decided someone needs to pay damages, such as resulting from a lawsuit.

It is very common for a health insurance company to receive claims for someone who has been in an automobile accident. Providers will often have you fill out some kind of form that asks you if your injuries are the result of an accident. This is why they do that. The provider is much more likely to get paid if they submit the bill to the right place from the beginning.

Coordination of Benefits

Coordination of benefits (COB) is needed when health insurance benefits are available to you from multiple sources. The case where spouses are covered by their own as well as their spouse's insurance is rarely seen today. To help control costs, most companies do not allow spousal coverage if insurance is available to the spouse from their own employer. But this used to be a common practice and requires coordination of benefits, and there are still some situations where benefits are payable from multiple sources, such as children being insured on both parent's plans.

Coordination of benefits is the process of understanding the multiple sources that exist, understanding what the other plan or plans pay, and making payments according to the plans' provisions for COB. If there is only one source of health insurance then there is no coordination of benefits, because there is no other health insurance plan to coordinate with.

The administrator of your health insurance might not know that you are covered by multiple sources. They may ask you this question when you enroll or at a later time, such as when they are processing a claim and suspect that other insurance may exist.

Explanation of Benefits (EOB)

When your health insurance claim is processed by an insurance company or administrator, they must send you something called an explanation of benefits. As the title suggests, it is an explanation of how benefits have been applied to the processing of the claim. It contains very detailed information about charges, discounts, the available benefit, amounts applied to deductible and OOP, and the payment that has been made to a provider (if any). The EOB must also contain the process for appealing the decisions made in processing the claim if there is any full or partial denial of benefits. Often, EOBs are available both as a paper and electronic copy.

> *Often, people believe the EOB is a bill. It is NOT a bill. It is usually printed right on the EOB "THIS IS NOT A BILL", but people still become confused. It is simply an explanation of the decisions made in processing the claim. If you owe the provider's office something, the provider's office will send you a bill. The EOB is sent by whoever has processed the claim.* You should never need to make a payment directly to the insurance company or administrator for medical services you have received.

HIPAA

If you have visited a provider at any point since 1996, you have probably signed a HIPAA form. HIPAA is short for the Health Insurance Portability and Accountability Act of 1996. It is a set of rules that, among other things, control the use and disclosure of your health information—called protected health information (PHI) — by individuals and organizations. It gives you privacy rights to understand and control how your health information is used. The goals of the privacy rule are to assure that your health information is properly protected while allowing the flow of health information needed to provide and promote high-quality healthcare and to protect the public's health and well-being. The act balances permitting important uses of information while protecting the privacy of people receiving medical care (HHS.gov, 2013).

Any time you seek medical treatment from a healthcare professional, you will be asked to sign a HIPAA form that explains your rights, and also asks if there is anyone other than you whom they can speak to about your care. If you do not list anyone, they cannot legally discuss your medical condition or treatment with anyone except you. You have the right under this law to be the only one who they can share your health-related information with.

HIPAA does not apply to other medical professionals or outside organizations (insurance companies, labs, etc.) that may need the information to assist with the treatment you are receiving, however it specifies that only the bare minimum information should be shared, to perform the function they are performing. For example, an entity who needs information for billing should not be sent detailed information about your diagnosis. And parents/guardians will not be denied condition or treatment information about their minor children. Anyone who handles your information is subject to the guidelines in the HIPAA act. They must protect your PHI and only disclose it when, and only as much as necessary to aid in your medical treatment. You will find at some point, as you talk to a hospital or provider's office about a relative or friend, that you are denied information because you are not on the patient's HIPAA list.

HIPAA is taken very seriously in the healthcare and health insurance industries. There are very serious penalties for not protecting PHI.

Examples:

The following examples will help illustrate some of the concepts we just discussed. Each example specifies how the plan is setup for that scenario. Be aware that your plan may differ from these examples.

Example 1: Your plan pays eighty percent after a $500 deductible is met for services provided by an in-network provider. In this example, you have not met your deductible or your OOP.

1. A provider performs a procedure on you in his office and charges $800 for the office visit and the procedure.

2. The provider's office creates a claim and sends it to the administrator for your health insurance plan.

3. The administrator says, "Wait a minute, that's more than the provider's contract with the network allows him to charge for those services. The provider must accept $300." ($200 for the procedure in his office and $100 for the office visit). $500 is the network discount amount, and $300 is the allowable charge for the procedure and the office visit.

4. The administrator looks at your records to determine how full your deductible and OOP buckets are, and what benefits your plan has. The administrator determines that the procedure is covered, it applies to your deductible, and your plan has twenty percent coinsurance after your deductible has been met.

5. Your deductible bucket is not yet full, so the administrator begins to fill it with what you are being charged by the provider. Your $500 deductible bucket currently contains $300. $200 will be put into your deductible bucket, completely filling the bucket. (Your plan's $500 deductible has been met.) There is still $100 of the $300 charge remaining ($300 - $200 = $100). Of that $100,

the insurer will pay eighty percent, because the plan has twenty percent coinsurance. That amount is eighty dollars. You are responsible for the amount that fits in the deductible bucket plus your twenty percent coinsurance, or a total of $220.

6. The administrator pays the provider eighty dollars and sends them an EOP explaining the payment. The administrator sends you an EOB explaining how the claim has been processed, the charges, the discounts, any amounts that have been applied to any of your buckets, and how much has been paid to the provider.

7. The provider sees $800 charged, $300 allowed, and also a payment from the insurer for eighty dollars. So, the provider sends you a bill for $220 so they can collect the full $300 they are allowed.

8. When you pay the provider's bill, the provider will have the full $300 that he has been allowed to charge; the eighty dollars from the insurer and $220 from you. He writes off the $500 he was not allowed to charge.

9. The $220 that you have paid to the provider is all out-of-pocket. The administrator puts as much of the $220 into your OOP bucket as will fit.

Example 2: Your plan pays eighty percent after a $500 deductible is met for services provided by an in-network provider. In this example, you have met your deductible but not your OOP.

1. A provider performs a procedure on you in his office and charges $800 for the office visit and the procedure

2. The provider's office creates a claim and sends it to the administrator for your health insurance plan.

3. The administrator says, "Wait a minute. That's more than the provider's contract with the network allows him to charge. He

can only charge $200 for that procedure in his office and $100 for the office visit." $500 is the network discount amount and $300 is the allowable charge for the procedure and the office visit.

4. The administrator looks at your records to determine how full your deductible and OOP buckets are and what benefits your plan has. The administrator determines that the procedure is covered, it applies to your deductible, and your plan has twenty percent coinsurance after the deductible has been met.

5. Your deductible bucket is already full, so the $500 plan deductible has already been met, and no more deductible can be put into your deductible bucket. The insurer will pay eighty percent of the entire allowed amount, because the plan has twenty percent coinsurance. That amount is $240.

6. The administrator pays the provider $240 and sends the provider an EOP explaining how the payment has been calculated. The administrator sends you an EOB explaining how the claim has been processed, the charges, the discounts, any amounts that have been applied to any of your buckets, and how much they have paid the provider.

7. The provider sees $800 charged, $300 allowed, and also a payment from the insurer of $240. The provider sends you a bill for sixty dollars (the amount of your coinsurance), which is the balance remaining on your $300 bill.

8. When you pay the provider's bill, the provider will have the full $300 that he has been allowed to charge. $240 from the insurer, and sixty dollars from you. He will write off the $500 he has not been allowed to charge.

9. The sixty dollars that you have paid the provider is all out-of-pocket. The administrator will put the entire sixty dollars into your OOP bucket.

Example 3: Your plan pays eighty percent after a $500 deductible is met for services provided by an in-network provider. In this example, you have met your deductible and your OOP.

1. A provider performs a procedure on you in his office and charges $800 for the office visit and the procedure.

2. The provider's office creates a claim and sends it to the administrator of your health insurance plan.

3. The administrator says, "Wait a minute. That's more than the provider's contract with the network allows him to charge. He can only charge $200 for that procedure in his office and $100 for the office visit." $500 is the network discount amount and $300 is the allowable charge.

4. The administrator looks at your records to determine how full your deductible and OOP buckets are, and what benefits your plan has. The administrator determines the procedure is covered, it applies to your deductible, and your plan has twenty percent coinsurance after the deductible has been met.

5. Your deductible bucket is already full, so the $500 plan deductible has been met, and no more deductible can be put into your deductible bucket.

6. Your OOP bucket is *also* full. According to your plan, you should no longer have any out-of-pocket expenses during this plan year and because of that, the insurer will pay one hundred percent of the allowable.

7. The administrator pays the provider $300 and sends the provider an EOP explaining the payment. The administrator sends you an EOB explaining how the claim has been processed, the charges, the discounts, any amounts that have been applied to any of your buckets, and how much they have paid the provider.

8. The provider sees $800 charged, $300 allowed, and also a payment from the insurer for $300, and your bill is considered paid-in-full. The provider does not bill you. He writes off the $500 he was not allowed to charge.

Example 4: Your plan pays eighty percent after a $500 deductible is met for services provided by an in-network provider and you have a twenty-dollar copay. Deductible does not apply. (Copays do not apply to deductible or OOP). In this example, you have not met your deductible

1. A provider performs a procedure on you in his office and charges $800 for the procedure and the office visit. The receptionist collects a twenty-dollar copay from you before the procedure to pay for the office visit

2. The provider's office creates a claim and sends it to the administrator of your health insurance plan.

3. The administrator says, "Wait a minute. That's more than the provider's contract with the network allows him to charge. He can only charge $200 for that procedure in his office and $100 for the office visit." $500 is the network discount amount and $300 is the allowable charge.

4. The administrator looks at your records to determine how full your deductible and OOP buckets are, and what benefits your plan has. The administrator determines the procedure is covered, it does *not* apply to the deductible, and there is a twenty-dollar copay for the office visit. The administrator also sees that you already paid a twenty-dollar copay to the provider for the office visit.

5. Since deductible does not apply, it does not matter how full your deductible bucket is, and the twenty-dollar copay you paid to the provider is not added to the deductible bucket because your plan says copays do not apply to the deductible.

6. There is still a $280 balance on the provider's allowed charges after the twenty-dollar copay you paid. The administrator will pay the entire balance and pays the provider $280, and sends them an EOP explaining the payment. (Since deductible does not apply, the administrator pays one hundred percent of the charge. The twenty-dollar copay is your entire responsibility for the office visit and the remainder is paid by the insurer).

7. The administrator sends you an EOB explaining how the claim has been processed, the charges, the discounts, any amounts applied to any of your buckets, and how much they have paid the provider.

8. The provider sees $800 charged, $300 allowed, and that you paid a twenty-dollar copay. The provider now has your twenty-dollar copay, and the $280 from the insurer and they have been paid in full. The provider does not bill you.

9. Since the twenty-dollar copay does not apply to the OOP, nothing is added to the OOP bucket.

Example 5: Your plan pays fifty percent after a $1500 deductible is met for services provided by an out-of-network provider. *In this example, you have not met your out-of-network deductible, and you use an out-of-network provider.*

1. An out-of-network provider performs a procedure on you in his office and charges $800 for the procedure and office visit.

2. The provider's office creates a claim and sends it to the administrator of your health insurance plan.

3. The administrator sees that it is an out-of-network provider. *No discount is allowed or applied to the $800 charge because the provider does not have a contract with your network.*

4. The administrator looks at your records to determine how full your deductible and OOP buckets are, and what benefits your

plan has. The administrator determines the procedure is covered, and it applies to your deductible. Your plan has fifty percent coinsurance (for out-of-network providers) after your out-of-network deductible is met. (That's right, there is a new bucket to hold the out-of-network deductible and it's *much* larger than your in-network deductible bucket.) Since this is an out-of-network provider, they have no contractual obligation to accept a discounted amount. But that doesn't mean you will always pay what is billed. The administrator determines the allowable charge for the procedure by applying the plan's eighty percent of UCR rule. According to your plan, they will pay fifty percent, but the insurer determines what is allowable, just like if a network was forcing a discount. The UCR for this procedure (and office visit) in your area is only $500. The allowable amount for this charge is eighty percent of $500, or $400. This is the amount the administrator will use for the remainder of the claims processing as the allowable charge.

5. Your much larger out-of-network deductible bucket is not full so it begins to fill it with the $400. You have only met $100 of your $1500 out-of-network deductible. It is able to get the entire $400 into the deductible bucket without it being full. The $400 is also placed into the much larger out-of-network OOP bucket. Since the entire allowable amount is placed into your deductible bucket, the insurer pays none of the charges.

   Note: Sometimes these amounts will also go into your in-network deductible and OOP buckets depending on how your plan is structured.

6. The administrator does not send a payment to the provider, but does send an EOP explaining why they are not making any payment on the claim. The administrator sends you an EOB explaining the allowable amount, and that all of the allowable amount has been applied to your deductible.

7. The provider sees $800 charged and $400 allowed and that they received no payment from the insurer. The provider can accept

the allowable amount and bill you $400, but may try to get you to pay the entire $800 charge, or something in-between. You can see how costly it can be to use an out-of-network provider. If you are charged the entire $800, this might be a good time to put those negotiating skills to use to see what the provider is willing to accept.

8. If your out-of-network deductible bucket had been full, and the administrator could not get any more money into it, then your plan says there is fifty percent coinsurance. In that case, the administrator would have sent the provider $200 and the provider would have had the same options. Bill you the difference between the allowable and what the insurer paid ($200), or try to charge you the $600 remaining on his full charge.

CHAPTER 10

Precertification

Precertification is sometimes referred to as preauthorization, prenotification, or prior authorization or approval. This chapter explains the meaning of the term, and how the precertification process is used to help control healthcare and health insurance costs.

Determining Medical Necessity

You may also see terms like utilization review (UR) and utilization management (UM). While these terms, and the terms above all have slightly different meanings, for purposes of this guide, we are going to lump them all together and focus on what is referred to as medical necessity.

According to the Utilization Review Accreditation Commission (URAC), an accreditor of healthcare organizations, utilization management (UM) is "the evaluation of the medical necessity, appropriateness, and efficiency of the use of healthcare services, procedures, and facilities under the provisions of the applicable health benefits plan, sometimes called 'utilization review'" (NAIC, 2010) UR/UM is the processes a company uses to determine if the planned services are appropriate. Precertification or preauthorization is what the provider and/or member is responsible for doing before receiving services that require preauthorization.

Utilization Management is a process where your insurer, administrator, or someone they hire to perform this function makes a decision about whether a healthcare service, treatment plan, or prescription drug is medically necessary. That means it is necessary and appropriate for whatever condition it is being used to treat. This process is performed before the service is provided to you.

Your health insurance plan may require preauthorization for certain services or drugs before you receive them. This requirement is often waived if it is an emergency situation

Employers and other insurers want to make sure you get the right care at the right time, and that your care does not cost them—or you— more than it should. Trained medical professionals (such as registered nurses) review the medical necessity and appropriate use of healthcare services. To determine the medical necessity, they compare the planned treatment to industry standards for care. They *do not* determine if benefits are payable under your health insurance plan.

If your health insurance plan does not recognize something as medically necessary and you elect to move forward with the treatment, then it could lower the amount of money the insurer will pay. Your plan may provide no reimbursement for the service if required preauthorization is not obtained. Some plans contain precertification penalties. Failure to obtain preauthorization for a procedure that requires one, may result in a penalty even if the claim is payable. Penalties are typically a set dollar amount ($300 - $500).

For example, in some cases, plastic surgery is considered medically necessary and is covered under a health insurance plan. In most cases, plastic surgery is not medically necessary and is not covered because it is seen as an elective procedure. Gastric bypass surgery is often only covered if it is medically necessary as well. This type of surgery could be an elective procedure in which case it will not be covered. Also, certain prescription drugs may not be considered medically necessary, for example, drugs used to treat fertility, weight loss, or weight gain, among many others. Be aware that most health insurance plans contain some kind of preauthorization requirement.

> *It is very important that you understand what procedures your plan says require preauthorization. Failure to obtain a preauthorization could result in your entire claim being DENIED. Often, preauthorization is obtained by the provider, but you should understand what the requirement is, and verify that it has been carried out. Ask your provider who is doing preauthorization.*

Preauthorization is not a guarantee of payment under your plan. This process determines medical necessity and appropriateness of care, but the procedure, treatment, or medication still needs to be covered under the plan in order for it to be covered.

> *For complex procedures or other expensive treatments, it is important to verify benefits as well as complying with any precertification requirements of your plan.*

Here is an example of what could happen:

A woman was diagnosed with Severe Crohn's disease. She was prescribed an oral medication but after several weeks it was obvious that she needed more aggressive treatment. She was prescribed infusion therapy with Remicade. Because of the cost of this treatment, the doctor and the woman both contacted her insurance to get the procedure pre-authorized. After some back-and-forth, the insurer agreed that the therapy was medically necessary. She felt good about complying with the requirements of her plan and she began the treatment. After a few weeks, she received an EOB that said her claim was denied because the treatment was not covered as part of her health insurance plan's benefits. She soon received a bill for $21,000 for one infusion. At that point she had already had three infusions. Assuming the same thing was going to happen with the other two infusions, she contacted her insurer. The insurer's response was, "Just because we approved the medicine, doesn't mean it's covered." She received bills for a total of $64,000.

Predetermination (Identifying the Level of Benefits)

The predetermination of benefits documents and communicates the specifics of coverage. A predetermination from the insurer includes information regarding the services that are covered, and to what level, how the insurer will pay the claim, and when you or your provider will receive payment. A predetermination is often obtained before expensive dental procedures because dental coverage is often limited. Predetermination does not always occur, and is not really part of utilization management, but is included here since it is often confused with preauthorization. A predetermination is not usually performed unless requested by you or your provider.

CHAPTER 11

Appeals

In this chapter, you will learn about your right to appeal (disagree with) a decision that has been made by your insurer if you believe the decision was made in error. Plans may have different processes for appealing decisions, but your right to appeal and certain minimum requirements that must be met by the process are set by state or federal regulations.

In an earlier chapter of this guide, you learned that all the moving parts had to work together perfectly for the process to be successful. Unfortunately, the parts often *do not* work together harmoniously. The first step for you is selecting the plan that is best for you. But the first step in the life of a health insurance claim occurs at the provider's office where they create the claim with the information about you and the services provided to you. In an earlier chapter that discusses claim processing, you read that claims often contain errors, in part because of the thousands of combinations of codes that can be used. It is difficult to know how often claims actually contain errors. But the fact is that errors on claims are prevalent, and if this first step is not done properly, you cannot expect the rest of the process to be accurate. As a consumer, you are most likely not going to have any idea of what the problem is when an error is made.

Imagine any of the following realistic scenarios:

- You receive some medical treatment that you think should be covered by your health insurance plan, and then you receive a bunch of bills from one or more providers or facilities that you are not expecting. And you are sure the people involved with your treatment are in-network.
- A provider determines that your health requires you to have a certain treatment, and the insurer determines that it is not medically necessary before you have the treatment. They inform you that they will not pay for it. But you and your provider disagree with the insurer's decision.
- You are told by your insurer that a particular prescription medicine is not covered under your health insurance plan, but you think it should be.
- Your health insurance coverage has been canceled by the insurer altogether.

Being blind-sided by any of these situations could be scary and potentially have a significant financial or emotional impact on your life, especially if you are ill and hoping the medical treatment or medication will reduce or eliminate symptoms, and you are assuming (or have been told) it will be covered by your insurance plan. The insurer's first decision is not final. You have a right to appeal certain decisions that have been made that are not in your favor.

Statistics on the denial rate for claims, and the appeal success rate vary widely across insurance carriers. The thing that has remained consistent across all studies is that consumers rarely appeal denied claims. A Kaiser Foundation report in 2019 says that of 41 million denied claims examined, consumers appealed fewer than 200,000. That represents an appeal rate of less than one-half of one percent. (Pollitz, Cox, & Fehr, 2019).

A Kaiser Foundation report in 2021 states [O]n average, appeals resulted in a reversal of the initial denial in fourteen percent of cases, though with wide variations among individual insurers, which had reversal rates ranging from one percent to eighty-eight percent. It later says consumers rarely appeal claims denials to their issuers, and when they do, issuers usually uphold their original decision. In 2019, HealthCare.gov consumers appealed just over one-tenth of one percent of denied in-network claims, and issuers upheld sixty percent of those appeals. (Karen Pollitz, 2021)

Many federal laws exist to protect members and attempt to simplify the insurance process. Federal laws say that employee health insurance plans need to contain claims procedures that are reasonable, and include a process of notifying claimants about the determination of benefits in a reasonable amount of time. If all or part of a claim is denied, the claimant must be notified in a reasonable amount of time but no longer than ninety days after receipt of the claim. The notification has to include specific reasons for the denial. The laws also state that "[e]very employee benefit plan shall establish and maintain a procedure by which a claimant shall have a reasonable opportunity to appeal an adverse benefit determination to a fiduciary of the plan, and under which there will be a full and fair review of the claim and the adverse benefit determination." It also states that the right to appeal and the procedure to use must be documented in the plan's documents, as well as accompanying the notification of denial. (29 CFR § 2560.503-1 - Claims procedure., 2020)

There are specific kinds of adverse benefit determinations (denials) that can be appealed. Sometimes the insurance company or administrator determines that you are not eligible to receive a certain benefit. When this occurs, you receive an EOB or a letter that says all or part of your medical claim has been denied. This is also reflected in an

EOP sent to the provider, which results in the provider balance billing you. According to HealthCare.gov, these are the reasons for denial that you can appeal:

- The benefit isn't offered under your health plan
- Your medical problem began before you joined the plan
- You have received health services from an out-of-network provider
- The requested service or treatment is "not medically necessary"
- The requested service or treatment is an "experimental" or "investigative" treatment
- You're no longer enrolled or eligible to be enrolled in the health plan
- They are revoking or canceling your coverage going back to the day you originally enrolled claiming you gave false or incomplete information when you applied for coverage

Source: (CMS.gov, 2020)

Many states have health insurance consumer advocates that you can contact to help with an appeal. FamiliesUSA.org offers a list of state resources. Another good resource is the nonprofit Patient Advocate Foundation, which handles health-insurance appeals for free. If you are not comfortable with either of those options, numerous private healthcare advocacy organizations will assist you with an appeal. Some of these groups will also help you negotiate a lower payment for large provider bills.

Filing an appeal is not an easy process, and not always the appropriate first course of action. If you have a complaint about your health insurance plan that does not involve a specific treatment denial, you can file a complaint or grievance with your insurer or administrator. *This is not considered an appeal.* Your plan will have specific instructions about how to file a grievance or complaint. Also, some denials are the result of simple errors made by the provider or the insurance company or even the claimant themselves that may be able to be corrected outside the formal appeal process with a few phone calls. Either you or your provider can contact the insurance company or administrator to request a reconsideration of a denial.

An appeal is a very specific request that you make of your insurer using a documented appeal process. You can appeal a decision made by your insurer or administrator through an "internal appeal" where you ask your insurance company or administrator to do a full and fair review of its decision.

Providers cannot appeal on your behalf. The provider can call the insurer with questions or complaints, but only the insured can officially appeal a benefit determination and start the formal appeal process.

If your insurer or administrator still denies payment or coverage, the law permits you to have an independent third party review the plan's decision. This final process is often referred to as an "external review". Some group plans may require more than one level of internal review before you can request an external review.

Appeal procedures generally contain very specific rules about how and when things need to occur. Federal laws require that an appeal procedure give the claimant at least 180 days to file an appeal. But there are strict deadlines for every step of every level of appeal. After your insurance company reviews your appeal and reconsiders its decision(s), they are required to explain their decision and let you know how you can disagree with its decision, if you still do not agree.

i

> *If your appeal is related to treatment that is urgent, then by law, the appeal process must be expedited. An urgent condition is one in which your health may be in serious jeopardy, or in the opinion of your physician, you may experience pain that cannot be adequately controlled while you wait for a decision on your appeal.*

Internal Review:

The purpose of the internal review is to determine if your claim or request for preauthorization has been processed correctly. You may ask your insurer to conduct a full and fair review of its decision, and your claim will be reviewed by someone new who looks at all the information submitted and consults with qualified medical professionals if necessary. This reviewer cannot be the same person who has made the initial decision, and the reviewer cannot use the original denial as a basis for their decision.

External Review:

If your appeal is denied after an internal review, you have the right to take your appeal to an independent third party for review. This is called an external review. In this step, the insurer no longer gets the final say over whether to pay a claim.

The Affordable Care Act requires that health insurance plans provide for external review of claim denials by an independent party. Depending on whether the plan is fully-insured or self-insured the requirements are slightly different. One of the main differences is, for fully-insured plans, the claimant can reach out directly to a third-party reviewer. In the case of self-insured plans, you are entitled to an external review, but the insurer selects the reviewer. The external review will be handled by an independent review organization (IRO) who has been accredited by URAC.

> *If your health insurance plan is self-insured, you may be able to get some help from your HR department. They cannot show favoritism toward you over other employees. But since they are self-insured, and it is their funds that are being questioned, they may be willing to get involved.*

Marketplace Appeal

According to HealthCare.gov, if you don't agree with a decision made by the health insurance marketplace, you may be able to file an appeal. These are decisions that are made before you even enroll in a plan. You can appeal the following kinds of marketplace decisions made when trying to enroll in one of the plans:

- Whether you're eligible to buy a marketplace plan, including a catastrophic health insurance plan
- Whether you can enroll in a marketplace plan outside the regular open enrollment period
- Whether you're eligible for lower costs based on your income
- The amount of savings you're eligible for
- A reduction in the amount of savings you are eligible for
- Whether you're eligible for Medicaid or the Children's Health Insurance Program (CHIP). (Note: This applies only in certain states where the federally facilitated Marketplace makes the Medicaid eligibility determination).

Source: (HealthCare.gov, 2020)

Medicare appeal

Medicare claims have an entirely different appeals process. You can appeal if Medicare or your Medicare Advantage plan denies your benefit(s).

The appeal process has five levels. If you disagree with the decision made at any level of the process, you can generally go to the next level. At each level, you'll get instructions in the decision letter on how to move to the next level of appeal. Appeals for original Medicare are initiated by contacting whoever pays the Medicare claims and their contact information can be found on your Medicare summary notice (MSN). For Medicare Advantage and Part D plans, you initiate your claim appeal through the company who issues the plan.

CHAPTER 12

COBRA

If you have insurance and then for whatever reason you are no longer covered, (such as becoming unemployed, or removed from a spouse's coverage), you will benefit from what you learn in this chapter about COBRA coverage.

COBRA stands for the Consolidated Omnibus Budget Reconciliation Act of 1985. This federal act requires employer-sponsored group health insurance plans to allow you and your covered dependents to continue your group coverage for a specific number of months after a qualifying event that causes the loss of your group health insurance coverage. Qualifying events include reduced work hours, termination of employment, a child becoming an over-age dependent, Medicare eligibility, or death or divorce of a covered employee. Like Medicare, COBRA is complex and has many rules. This guide provides an introduction and overview of COBRA.

Employers are required to explain employees' COBRA rights and rates when the employee first joins the company, as well as when a qualifying event occurs. This communication is called a "Cobra notice" or "Cobra rights notice". The Cobra notice is long and complex and most likely ignored. But if you have a qualifying event, it is important to review the Cobra Notice that you are sent to ensure you understand your rights.

If you have a qualifying event that makes you eligible for COBRA coverage, your employer must give you at least sixty days to decide if you want to enroll in COBRA. This is called the election period. Technically, the employer has thirty days to notify the administrator of a qualifying event and the administrator then has fourteen days to mail out the Cobra notice. The sixty-day election period window begins on the date you are notified of your COBRA rights. If you notify your employer (or whoever is doing the COBRA administration) that you want to elect COBRA during the election period, then the coverage is retroactive to the date of the qualifying event, although you must still pay any premiums that have been missed during that time.

> *If you know that your gap in coverage is going to be less than the election period, you can wait and see if anything happens during that period that will necessitate health coverage and then make your election.*

In most cases, you are allowed to continue COBRA coverage for eighteen months; however, there are a few special qualifying events that give employees the right to continue COBRA coverage for longer.

Does that sound too good to be true? The major drawback of COBRA is the cost. If you are employed and the qualifying event is the loss of your employment, here is the problem. While employed, your employer most likely has paid a portion (or all) of your health insurance premiums. The amount (if any) that was deducted from your pay each week to pay for health insurance was likely only a small portion of the premium. Once you separate from the employer, they will no longer pay their portion, and you are responsible for the entire premium. Even though you keep the same coverage you have had as an employee, it is no longer twenty or thirty dollars a week for your family coverage that has been taken from your paycheck.

In most cases, you cannot make changes to the coverage you have had as an employee, and there are certain cases where an employer can cancel your coverage, such as if they no longer offer health insurance to any of their employees. Whoever has been doing the administration for your health insurance plan while you were employed will most likely continue in that role. However, there may be a new party introduced that does the COBRA administration. That includes providing notices, doing your enrollment, performing customer service, and collecting your premium payments.

During the COVID-19 pandemic, many businesses have been forced out of business due to social distancing guidelines. If a business is no longer operating, a former employee cannot continue their coverage under COBRA. Also, anyone receiving COBRA benefits at the time the business closed will lose their benefits. People in either of the situations above became uninsured or forced to obtain insurance through the marketplace or other private sources.

CHAPTER 13

Other Benefits in Your Plan

Most health insurance plans contain benefits in addition to medical health insurance used for doctors and hospitals. This chapter explains some of the other benefits your health insurance plan may contain.

Prescription Medication Benefit

Most major medical health insurance plans will have some level of prescription drug coverage included. Most of the time, we treat illnesses and injuries with medication. So, it makes sense to tie a prescription drug benefit to a health insurance plan.

Pharmacy Benefit Managers (PBMs)

Prescription drugs are often the most widely used benefit in a health insurance plan and in many cases the most expensive. One of the items you will most likely see on your medical ID card is the pharmacy benefit manager. It will most likely be labeled "Rx," "pharmacy," or "prescriptions" instead of PBM.

The pharmacy portion of a health insurance benefit is extremely complex. Most insurers carve out that portion of healthcare to a PBM who handles everything related to prescriptions. Caremark, Express Scripts, and Magellan are examples of larger PBMs that you may have heard of. A PBM handles everything drug-related as part of the health insurance benefit but reports back to your plan's administrator. They are like an entirely separate insurer or administrator, but the benefits are contained in a comprehensive health insurance plan administered by your insurer or Administrator.

When you visit a pharmacy to have a prescription filled or to pick up a prescription called-in by your physician, you will need to provide your insurance ID card to the pharmacist like any other provider. The insurance ID card contains information about your PBM, including how to contact them. Your pharmacy will contact the PBM to determine if you are a member in good standing, if the particular medication is included in the benefits of your plan, and what percentage of the drug's cost you should be charged. The pharmacist will verify with your PBM that you are not trying to receive more medication than you are allowed, such as trying to refill a prescription too early. Most PBMs also offer mail-order services that are usually less costly to the consumer.

If necessary, the pharmacy (just like any provider) will submit a claim to the PBM and receive payment from the PBM just like a medical claim. The specifics about what you have been charged and what you have paid is sent to the TPA or insurer to be included in the out-of-pocket and deductible buckets (if required based on your particular plan). The PBM will send an EOB to you and EOP to the provider explaining how the pharmacy claim has been processed just like the insurer or administrator does for medical claims.

Rx Discount Cards

Despite continuing discussion in the US Congress, prescription drug prices are not regulated. Congress continues to debate the need for prescription drug price regulation. The cost of a prescription may differ significantly between pharmacies (just like the cost of medical procedures). Plus, the markups on any medication could be very large. Insurance companies have been passing more of the cost of medications on to patients in recent years. As you saw earlier in this handbook, there are some medications for treating rare disorders that could cost over ten thousand dollars per month, so the impact of medication cost can be substantial.

The cash prices (meaning non-health insurance prices) at pharmacies are usually very high. But if you can do a little research, great discounts can be found. Some pharmacies (usually grocery stores or big-box stores) offer very cheap cash prices for some generic drugs. Many pharmacies publish a list of generic drugs with cheap cash prices, with some even being free to their member customers.

Prescription discount cards provide a way for you to obtain lower-priced medications if you are paying in cash (as opposed to going through an insurance plan). There is no cost to use these cards, and they often provide discounts of eighty to ninety percent. The healthcare community understands that prescription medication plays a big part in prevention and treatment of health conditions. And therefore, access to prescription drugs is of major importance. Many different prescription discount cards are available and can be obtained at physicians' offices and clinics, and through the mail from most PBMs.

According to the website CostsofCare.org, an organization that specializes in helping clinicians and health systems deliver better care at lower cost, a PBM "sets up a network of participating pharmacies that agree to accept the cards. Then, the PBM negotiates with each pharmacy chain and all the participating local pharmacies to offer a discount on the drugs they dispense. The discount offered is usually a percentage of the cash price of the drug and the percentage may vary from drug to drug."

The article goes on to say, "The PBM does its best to negotiate the best discount from the pharmacies. Some PBMs do a better job of this than others. The size of the PBM, its market share, and how much business it will direct to the pharmacy are all important factors in the overall final discount" (Richard J. Sagall, 2013).

> *Beware of scams. You should never pay for a card or provide personal information to obtain one. Legitimate cards are free and contain a toll-free helpline that you can call with questions.*

Another thing to keep in mind is these cards can be great for those without insurance or prescription drug coverage, but if you have a health insurance plan that covers prescription medicine, drug copays with your insurance may be lower than using the discount card. If your prescription drug coverage has a deductible, the discount card might save you money before you meet your deductible, however; the price you pay will *not* go towards your deductible (into your deductible bucket) so it may offset.

Online and Mail-Order Pharmacies

Chances are, the PBM associated with your plan has a mail-order option for medications. It might be a mail-order pharmacy owned by your PBM, or it could be a third-party online pharmacy contracted by your PBM. Either way, it's convenient and often cheaper. Many plans offer three months of medications for only two copays instead of three if you use their mail-order service.

As consumers turn more and more to the Internet to shop, they discover that there are an abundance of sites offering "low-cost" medications. Some are legitimate, and some not so much. Our email accounts are bombarded with advertisements for low-cost drugs. Many of the pharmacies state that they are free of U.S. regulation because they are not located in the United States, and no prescription is required.

i

> *Current U.S. laws do not allow citizens to purchase low-cost drugs in a foreign country and bring them into the United States. This includes Canada or Mexico, even though these countries often have the same drugs that are legally approved and licensed in the United States, at a much lower cost.*
>
> *This law is rarely enforced.*
>
> *The Trump administration tried to make it legal for pharmacies to import drugs from other countries. But ran into resistance from the US pharmaceutical industry who claim their opposition is to ensure that counterfeit drugs are kept out of the U.S. market. However, these efforts continue.*

In addition to being illegal to obtain prescription drugs without a prescription, some online pharmacies pose a serious health threat, selling unapproved, counterfeit, and potentially unsafe drugs to consumers. According to the United States Food and Drug Administration (FDA), only three percent of online pharmacies reviewed by the National Association of Boards of Pharmacy are in compliance with U.S. pharmacy laws and practice standards (FDA.gov, 2018).

Maybe you are reading this, and you think it's worth the risk to save the money. Be aware that drugs from other countries are manufactured with an entirely different set of standards than U.S. drug companies. Medications you receive from outside the country might have too much or too little of the active ingredient you need to treat your disease or condition. It's also possible that the drug could contain the wrong ingredient completely. It could be ineffective, or it could be dangerous or even deadly. Sometimes, there are translation issues, or differences in meaning in other countries.

A perfect example is prostate medication Flomax. In the United States, Flomax is the brand name of the drug tamsulosin. However, in

Italy, Flomax is an anti-inflammatory drug called morniflumate. There could be other examples that have more severe consequences.

If you plan to use an online pharmacy not affiliated with your insurance plan or PBM, there are a few things to look out for. Pharmacies that claim you can obtain medications without a prescription, are located outside the United States or ship worldwide, or send spam or unsolicited email offering cheap medications are not legitimate pharmacies and should be avoided. Here are some ways to identify a safe online pharmacy:

- Require a valid prescription from a doctor or another licensed healthcare professional.

- Are licensed by your state board of pharmacy or equivalent state agency (To verify the licensing status of a pharmacy, check your state board of pharmacy.)

- Have a U.S. state-licensed pharmacist available to answer your questions.

- Are in the United States, and provide a street address.

Source: (fda.gov, 2018)

Another way to identify a legitimate online pharmacy is to look for the National Association of Boards of Pharmacy's (NABP) Verified Internet Pharmacy Practice Sites seal, also known as the VIPPS® Seal. This seal means that the Internet pharmacy is safe to use because it has met state licensure requirements, as well as other NABP criteria.

Numerous resources will help identify or guide you to legitimate online pharmacies such as BuySafeRx.pharmacy. This is a website run by an organization called the Alliance for Safe Online Pharmacies (ASOP), whose mission is to combat illegal online pharmacies and counterfeit medicines.

Dental and Vision Benefits

Health insurance plans often contain some level of dental or vision benefits. Dental and vision benefits can be part of a comprehensive health insurance plan, or they could be stand-alone plans offered and purchased separately. Compared with medical health insurance plans, dental and vision insurance plans are much more straight forward, are easier to understand, and have lower premiums.

Dental Insurance

Dental benefits usually cover one or more of the following categories of services: preventative, basic procedures, major procedures, and orthodontics.

Most dental insurance plans cover preventive care, like cleanings and check-ups with no or minimal out-of-pocket costs to you. Dental plans usually cover an exam and cleaning every six months, and x-rays every year or 18 months, sometimes with no out-of-pocket cost to you.

Expenses related to other dental procedures—such as cavity fillings, annual X-rays, root canals, and other treatments—are often covered but subject to a deductible and copay or coinsurance. These kinds of services will fall into the "basic procedures" category of services, and most dental plans cover seventy to eighty percent of these procedures (after a deductible is satisfied), with you paying the remainder. Often, more expensive or elective procedures like whitening are not covered at all because they are not considered medically necessary. Medical necessity is much easier to determine in the case of dental benefits.

Dental plans often have annual maximums for certain benefits, or the entire dental benefit might be capped at a certain dollar level, like $1,500. Orthodontics, if covered at all, are usually not covered completely, and there's generally a separate lifetime and possibly yearly maximum specifically for orthodontic costs. Major procedures—such as crowns, bridges, inlays and dentures—if covered, are typically only minimally covered, with you paying more out-of-pocket expenses than other procedures.

Every plan differs in how procedures are categorized as preventive, basic, and major, so it is important to understand what is covered when comparing plans. Some plans group root canals as major procedures, while others treat them as basic procedures and cover much more of the cost.

Most plans follow a 100-80-50 coverage structure or something similar. That means they cover preventive care at one hundred percent, basic procedures at eighty percent, and major procedures at fifty percent. But a dental plan may elect not to cover some procedures, such as sealants, at all. As with any other type of insurance, higher levels of benefits mean higher premiums.

> *Medicare does not cover dental procedures, and if your Medicaid plan contains any dental benefits at all, it will only be for children.*

If you need a major procedure, you can ask your dentist to submit a pre-treatment estimate (predetermination). This will help you know what you'll likely owe out of pocket for the procedure.

> *Dental or other oral procedures that result from an injury may be covered by your medical insurance. Make sure you understand your medical and dental benefits.*

Like medical health insurance, dental insurance plans come in a variety of plan types.

- **preferred provider organization (PPO) plan:** Just like medical health insurance plans, dental PPO plans have a list of dentists who are members of a particular network and have agreed to accept discounted amounts for their services. If you have a PPO dental plan, charges from out-of-network dentists will be higher, and the benefits your plan pays will most likely be lower.

- **dental health maintenance organization (DHMO) plan:** Like a medical HMO, these plans have a network of dentists that accept a discounted fee like a PPO for members of their network. However, charges from an out-of-network dentist might not be covered at all.

- **discount dental plan**: This is a plan in which you get a discount on dental services from certain dentists who have agreed to provide this discount, and there are no claims.

- **dental savings plan**: Since dental expenses are so low compared with health-related care, some employers fund a savings account for each employee that can be used for any dental expense, for instance, $250 a year for each employee. Then the employee can see any provider, pay the costs out of pocket, and be reimbursed by the employer from the savings account.

Technically, discount plans and dental savings plans cannot even be called insurance because there is no policy involving cost sharing involved. When you have dental insurance and visit a provider, the provider bills the insurance company for the services they provide. You pay the provider any costs that are not covered under your plan (such as your deductible). But with a discount dental plan, the provider does not bill any insurance plan. Instead, you pay the provider directly, any amount that remains after the discount is applied. It's like having a coupon to use every time you visit the dentist.

During a routine dental exam, the dentist will be on the lookout for indications of other diseases. From a simple inspection of the inside of your mouth, a trained dentist can spot indication of ulcerative colitis, Crohn's disease, diabetes, HIV and other dangerous conditions. The dentist may want to perform additional tests if he suspects one of these conditions exist.

> *Beware of additional tests that the dentist recommends. Tests that go beyond what is considered a routine exam may involve additional costs that are not covered by your dental insurance plan.*

Vision

Vision insurance plan choices are very similar to medical and dental plans. The following types of plans are common:

- **preferred provider organization (PPO) plan**: Vision PPO plans have a list of vision providers who are members of a particular network and have agreed to accept discounted amounts for their services. If you have a PPO vision plan, charges from out-of-network providers will be higher, and the benefits your plan pays will most likely be lower.

- **health maintenance organization (HMO) plan:** Like a medical HMO, these plans have a network of vision providers that charge a discounted fee like a PPO for members of their network. However, charges from an out-of-network provider might not be covered at all.

- **indemnity vision insurance plan:** Like its medical counterpart, these plans will pay a fixed amount for different services and products. It might pay a fixed amount like $25 for a routine eye exam, and $100 for frames. A plan in this category might allow you to visit any provider.

- **discount vision insurance plan:** A discount plan like a dental discount plan simply provides a discount on products and services as long as you are using a vision provider who has agreed to accept this discount.

- **vision savings plans:** Like a dental savings plan, an employer may set up a special vision savings account and fund it for each employee. Then the employee can see any provider, pay the costs out of pocket, and be reimbursed by the employer from the savings account.

> *Beware: A routine and comprehensive eye exam may be different depending on how your provider defines them. They may have different levels of coverage in your vision insurance plan. Most insurance plans cover a routine eye exam that does not include additional tests. You may want to check what the provider's exam includes so you can understand what your insurance covers before visiting the provider.*

Vision insurance plans like dental plans often include a yearly or bi-yearly routine vision exam for a small copay, or no out of pocket expense to you. A routine eye exam usually includes tests for eye muscle movement, confirmation that your eyes can target moving objects, and visual acuity, which determines how well you can see letters on a chart. Several other tests can be performed during a routine eye exam that may or may not be covered by your insurance. A retinal exam is a common test that uses pupil dilation drops so the back of your eyes (your optic nerve head, retina, and retinal blood vessels) can be examined. Although relatively inexpensive, it is usually an additional charge that is sometimes not covered by your insurance plan.

A trained optometrist or ophthalmologist performing a routine eye exam can detect indications of major health problems, such as diabetes, high cholesterol, autoimmune disease, thyroid disease, and cancer. The person performing your exam may want to perform additional tests if he suspects one of these conditions exist.

> *Medicare does not provide any vision coverage; however, vision can be included as part of a Medicare Advantage plan.*

Elective procedures like LASIK are usually not covered by vision plans, although they may provide partial coverage. Treatment for glaucoma and cataracts are generally covered by your health insurance plan.

What is slightly different about vision insurance is that many people need corrective lenses (glasses or contacts), so you must purchase additional equipment that is usually only partially covered by the insurance plan. Vision plans usually pay for glasses and contacts up to a certain amount of money or provide a discount on frames, lenses, and contacts.

Telemedicine

Have you ever seen one of those old television shows where the town doctor comes to the house with his little black medical bag and treats little Johnny's fever? That actually used to occur, but it is pretty much ancient history now. And providers are too busy to sit on the telephone all day with you if you call with questions. Medical professionals realize it is often inconvenient to schedule an appointment and travel to see a provider, especially for minor illnesses like colds, fevers, or rashes. So, organizations have been created, staffed with licensed providers who can give you a diagnosis over the phone.

Something that has become very popular and has been getting a lot of attention recently is what is referred to as telemedicine, or telehealth. Especially since the COVID-19 pandemic required staying at home or social distancing. Think back to the last time you needed to see a doctor for something unexpected. Can you relate to this scenario? You are sick enough that you want to see your doctor, so you call the office and ask for an appointment. They tell you it is going to be three weeks until they can see you. That's hardly helpful if you have a fever and a stuffy nose *now*. They tell you if it's an emergency you can call 911. Those are your two options? Wait three weeks, or dial 911?

According to a 2017 study from Merritt Hawkins, the average wait time for a new doctor appointment is twenty-four days (Team, 2017). But let's say they *can* see you that day, or the next or even within a few days. You feel like you have won the lottery and you might even find yourself thinking, I hope I am still sick when my appointment occurs.

You take time off work, or maybe you are home already, but now you have to make yourself presentable to go out into the real world. You travel to the doctor's office, which may or may not be close to your house or work. And what if you have small children? You either need to find someone to watch them or go through the exercise of getting them ready to go out of the house. When you arrive at the doctor's office, you are told to take a seat and someone will be with you "shortly". And that "shortly" usually ends up being thirty minutes, an hour, or even more because—let's face it—doctor's rarely run on-schedule. And they shouldn't if they are taking the time to provide medical care to a variety of patients who are all completely different and have different needs. And what if you decide you can't wait the two or three days or a week to see your family doctor so you go to the emergency room or the urgent care, which is more expensive, and again, requires traveling and waiting?

This is the twenty-first century. What if there is a way to simply call a physician and be guaranteed to be seen (or heard) "shortly" and in this case it is only a reasonable wait time? With telemedicine, for a small fee, you can call one of these virtual providers and speak to a board-certified physician. You can use FaceTime, Skype, or Zoom to allow the provider to see your rash, pimple, or swollen whatever, or you can simply discuss your issues on the telephone. This is called a "virtual visit". If it is a minor issue, the physician may give you advice or even call in a prescription to a local pharmacy. For families with children, this service is great because it avoids having to run to the doctor constantly just to get a prescription for a runny nose. And we all know how often kids get sick. Depending on how your benefit plan is set up, the cost to you is less than seeing your family doctor, and the cost to the insurer is less as well. Its use is encouraged. Some employers even provide this to their employees at no cost because, in the long-run, it saves them money. Remember, if they are self-funded, they are paying your claims with their money. A fifty-dollar virtual visit beats a ninety-dollar office visit any day, for the person who is responsible for paying for it.

Studies have shown that the quality of care delivered by telemedicine is as effective as in-person care. And other studies have shown that patients who used telemedicine instead of conventional office visits had lower hospital re-admission rates. In an article in Healthcare IT News, Roy Schoenberg, MD—president and CEO of telehealth company American Well—said, "[E]nough time has passed that telemedicine technology vendors have gained the experience—and learned lessons from mistakes—so that the vendors are completely capable of providing safe and comprehensive care via technology" (Siwicki, 2016).

Unfortunately, there is a problem with awareness and utilization. People need to know it exists and, is available to them and to understand and recognize the benefits for the full benefit to be realized. That falls on the shoulders of the insurer. Insurers were required to offer telemedicine as part of their benefits once the pandemic struck. And telemedicine will most likely remain part of all plans in the future. And the awareness by insureds is likely to guarantee its continued use.

According to the Pew Research Center, the vast majority of Americans—ninety-six percent—now own a cellphone of some kind. And eighty-one percent of Americans now own a smartphone (Mobile Fact Sheet, 2019). We have the means to utilize this technology. Insurers need to push this hard as an option and something that they desire to see their members use by advertising the advantages. Although employees may not need to be pushed quite as hard after the pandemic.

What is the future of telemedicine? According to Roy Schoenberg in a FierceHealthcare.com article, "We've gotten good at targeting telehealth to younger, tech-savvier, affluent patients in their twenties, thirties, and forties. But we need to pay closer attention to where telehealth is needed most and can have a profound impact. Telehealth holds strong potential to help patients with serious and chronic conditions, such as cancer, diabetes and COPD, who typically require more frequent engagement to stay out of the hospital" (HealthcareStaff, 2019).

Healthcare Management

Healthcare management contains a variety of topics related to managing employees' health and thereby lowering healthcare-related costs for the employer and the employee. Two of those topics will be discussed in this section, wellness and case management. Wellness deals with preventative health measures helping employees stay well, maintain their health, and not need healthcare in the first place thus lowering healthcare costs. Case management occurs after someone is being treated for an illness or chronic condition and is sometimes referred to as disease management. Although these are not directly related to health insurance, they are often provided as part of a healthcare benefits package provided by employers. And they are often administered by the insurance company.

As you read this section, you may become alarmed that your employer has access to your medical records and things you would rather be kept private. You may fear that your health information could be used against you by your employer. Your participation in these programs and any information that is collected about your health are strictly regulated by HIPAA laws, just like any other PHI. Whoever has access to this information is strictly forbidden from sharing it with anyone whom you do not authorize, including your employer.

Wellness / Preventative Health Management

Most employers understand this premise: healthier employees = lower healthcare costs = lower premiums. Employers care about their employees. But they also care about their bottom-line. Healthier employees have less absenteeism, which results in greater productivity.

Many employers now offer some kind of wellness program and many offer wellness incentives like lower premiums, cash, or prizes for participating in wellness programs designed to improve health and promote a healthier lifestyle. Weight loss programs, stop-smoking programs, and fitness programs are just a few examples. Many larger companies have on-site gyms and exercise facilities. There are companies that provide healthcare management as a service, designing programs specific to a company's employees and, if necessary, becoming involved directly in the execution of the programs. These programs are often offered free of charge or for a significantly reduced cost to encourage participation.

In addition to wellness, these programs often begin with a comprehensive on-site employee health screening. Blood pressure and cholesterol screening and other tests create a snapshot of your current health. These results help predict your potential risk (or presence) for many conditions at their earliest, most treatable stages.

Someone with a medical background reviews your results, discusses the results with you, and notes any measurements that are significantly out-of-range. Employees with critical risk factors can be referred to their primary care physician for follow-up. It is human nature to want to avoid going to the doctor, and this may provide the encouragement that some people need or identify underlying health issues that will have otherwise gone unknown until it is too late.

Health coaching is sometimes offered to help with motivation or to help with questions. If you desire a more individualized wellness plan, you can contact a trained health coach who will work with you one-on-one to motivate and guide you toward healthier living.

Case Management / Disease Management

According to URAC, case management is "a collaborative process which assesses, plans, implements, coordinates, monitors, and evaluates options and services to meet an individual's health needs using communication and available resources to promote quality cost-effective outcomes" (NAIC, 2010). In this process, a Registered Nurse (RN) or other healthcare professional called a case manager will review your health situation and help plan and coordinate your care. They will act as your advocate, and assist you through the entire process of treatment and recovery. They will help identify appropriate providers and facilities while ensuring that available resources are being used in a timely and cost-effective manner. They may perform assessments regarding the level of care and make recommendations. They may help make sure you are taking your prescribed medication and following through with medical appointments. And they will provide assistance with insurance issues and education as well to help you be an informed consumer with lower levels of stress. Some illnesses are complex, and require complex treatment protocols that are difficult for most people and their families to understand. Case management nurses can help you and your family make informed decisions about your care.

Case Management opportunities are often identified during a hospitalization for a chronic, complex or large dollar situation. Or they could be identified during a review of claims. The RN works with the hospital's staff to assist in managing the case.

Disease management involves the management of chronic illnesses such as heart disease, diabetes, and cancer. Disease management, according to URAC, involves "a system of coordinated healthcare interventions and communications for populations with chronic conditions in which patient self-care efforts are significant" (NAIC, 2010). There are several components to disease management including patient education, monitoring, and communication with the patient, provider, and insurer or administrator. The goal of disease management is improving overall health of the person with a chronic illness. Disease management nurses are invaluable in helping the person receive successful treatment.

Healthcare Concierge

Healthcare concierge is not the same thing as concierge medicine described in chapter three. Healthcare concierge is a service that provides someone to be your healthcare/health insurance advocate, helping you navigate the complex healthcare and health insurance systems. It is included in some health insurance plans as an additional benefit. A healthcare concierge service can help you find in-network providers in your area and steer you away from providers who are out-of-network, help you understand your benefits, estimate costs, help you understand your EOB and even assist with filing an appeal.

Financial Wellness

In the beginning of the twenty-first century, insurers began realizing that your financial health can have a serious impact on your mental and physical health. If you are behind on your bills, have unpaid medical bills, are living paycheck-to-paycheck, are not paying your mortgage or rent, or have any other financial problems, you are probably feeling stressed and losing sleep, which has been shown to have a negative effect on your physical health. For that reason, some employers have begun incorporating programs to improve financial health into their benefits.

Financial health management could be in the form of one-on-one financial counseling, paycheck loans, help in learning to balance your checkbook, and investing, saving, or budgeting tips. Financial health and wellness could be part of an overall wellness program benefit.

Employee Assistance Program (EAP)

An employee assistance program offers free and confidential counseling and referrals to employees who have personal or work-related problems. Most EAPs address a broad range of issues that are known to have a negative impact on your mental and emotional health. Problems such as alcohol and other substance abuse, stress, grief, family problems, and psychological disorders. Most employers offer an EAP as part of employee's benefits.

CHAPTER 14

Traveling

People rarely think about health insurance in other countries if they are United States citizens. And this chapter will not explain health insurance worldwide. But there are several reasons that you should understand what happens if you are traveling outside the country and need medical care. This chapter will explain why this is important to know, and some of the preparations you can make before you travel.

You may need this information if you

- need medical treatment while traveling for business or pleasure,

- need medical treatment while temporarily living in another country,

- purposely travel outside the country for medical treatment.

If you are traveling outside the United States for any reason, you should research the healthcare system in your destination before you travel so you understand what healthcare is available and what your health insurance coverage will be. You cannot foresee illnesses or injuries, but if you are receiving treatment for some condition, you may want to wait until your treatment is complete before you travel.

Cruises pose a specific risk. If you become ill or are injured while on a cruise at sea, you may be able to wait until the next port of call or even wait for your return to the United States. But what if it is an emergency and you need to be flown off the ship back to the United States? According to the Centers for Disease Control (CDC), emergency evacuation by air-ambulance from a cruise ship can cost from $50,000 to $100,000. You may not even be covered by your domestic health insurance plan for receiving minor treatment aboard the ship which could end up being costly.

Most health insurance plans do not provide much, if any, coverage if you need medical care while outside the United States. And they will surely not cover the cost of being evacuated back to the United States for care. If you purchase trip health insurance, make sure it covers emergency evacuation

> *Medicare and Medicaid specifically do not provide any coverage at all outside the United States; however, a Medicare Advantage or Medigap plan may contain specific international coverage.*

If your insurance plan does not provide any out-of-country coverage, you will need to pay out of pocket and possibly will need to pay before you receive care. If you do have coverage, your health insurance plan will most surely treat any foreign providers as out-of-network. This means you will not receive any in-network discounts and your coinsurance share will be greater.

> *If you are traveling outside this country for any reason and you become ill, or are injured and need medical care, you can and should seek the help of the United States Embassy or Consulate in the country you are visiting. It is recommended that you know how to contact them before you travel.*

Traveling for Business or Pleasure

Before you travel, you can purchase supplemental travel insurance that will cover your medical costs while you are traveling outside the country. Travel insurance policies typically cover travel costs in case a trip is canceled or if you become ill and cannot travel, or lose your baggage. But some policies will cover medical expenses while you travel, and there are also stand-alone medical travel insurance policies that are specifically tailored toward medical expenses only. If you have purchased or are considering travel insurance, make sure you understand if they cover medical costs if you require medical care while traveling.

> *If you are traveling for business, you should contact your employer to find out if they provide any kind of benefit if you become ill or are injured while traveling for business purposes. If they do not provide any kind of benefits, you should ask them to reimburse you for the cost of obtaining travel insurance.*

A health insurance plan that provides coverage outside the United States may only provide coverage for a limited amount of time. If you are planning an extended stay outside the country, see the section below on living temporarily outside the United States.

If you purchase travel insurance, they will generally not cover any preexisting conditions. So be cautious if you have had a change in your medical condition within the last six months before you travel. And if you want to be extra cautious, you can research the healthcare system in the country you are traveling to, and even study local hospitals, clinics, and providers.

Even if you are covered by a domestic policy that provides full or partial coverage outside the country or have purchased some type of travel insurance, you still need to be prepared to pay all or a portion of the expenses up-front for medical care. Most foreign healthcare providers require payment in cash or by credit card before you are treated or admitted regardless of what insurance you carry.

Living Outside the United States Temporarily

If you plan to be out of the United States for an extended period but do not plan to become a permanent resident of the country you are visiting, a short-term travel insurance policy might not cover your needs. There may be a limit on how long they will cover you. Be sure to check with whoever issues the travel insurance to know for sure.

If this is the case, you may need to purchase a policy in the country you are visiting that covers you while you are there. If you are planning to do this and also plan to keep whatever insurance you have in the United States, you should check with your insurer to see if you are covered in case you need to be evacuated from that country to get medical care for a serious condition back in the United States. If not, you will want to make sure the policy you purchase locally contains provisions for that. You can purchase a global policy that covers you anywhere you travel, or a policy that only covers you in a specific country.

When purchasing a local health insurance policy, make sure the company providing the insurance is legitimate, and able to provide service levels that meet your needs. For instance, make sure they have a toll-free number that accesses English-speaking operators twenty-four hours per day. And it will be extremely helpful if they could help you locate nearby English-speaking medical providers and coordinate your care.

An American living in another country temporarily is called an America expatriate or expat as they are sometimes referred. Many companies offer expatriate health insurance plans. You can probably find a plan that covers pre-existing conditions, but you should beware that if you have dropped your domestic coverage in the United States, a foreign health insurance policy you purchase may not cover you in the United States if you have a need to return for medical treatment.

Canada and Mexico

Information on Canada and Mexico is included because of the proximity to the United States.

Canada's Universal Healthcare System

Canadian citizens can apply for public health insurance. Canada offers all citizens and permanent residents universal public health insurance, which affords low-cost access to private and public providers and facilities. Usually, you do not need to pay for most healthcare services. Unfortunately, expatriates with temporary residency in Canada are not eligible for the same benefits.

The health insurance program in Canada is called Medicare. But do not be confused because it has no association with United States Medicare. The insurance is funded through taxes. Government health insurance plans give you access to basic medical services, so citizens might also need private insurance to pay for things that government plans don't fully cover, like medication and dental and vision services.

There is sometimes a waiting period of up to three months to obtain insurance.

Each province or territory in Canada has its own health insurance plan with potentially different benefits. The plans are administered by the provincial and territorial ministries of health. You must show your ID card from the province where you live to obtain treatment; however, all provinces and territories will provide free emergency medical services, even if you don't have a government health card. There may be restrictions depending on your immigration status (Government of Canada, 2017).

Mexico's Public HealthCare System

In Mexico, there are two types of public healthcare coverage. The first and most common is the Instituto Mexicano del Seguro Social (IMSS), which is provided when you're employed full time with a Mexican company, regardless of your nationality. If you don't meet that criteria, you can purchase the same plan for a minimal premium.

With IMSS, the first year of coverage has limited benefits. Basically, the first year covers doctor's visits and emergencies. After the first year, the benefits are broader, including coverage for prescription drugs.

The second is called Seguro Popular. This insurance is provided by the Mexican government to ensure all Mexicans receive healthcare, regardless of their income or employment status. Seguro Popular is only applicable to those who aren't eligible for IMSS or private health insurance. The premiums are on a sliding scale, based on income and assets, and the poorest twenty percent do not pay a premium at all.

Expatriates are not eligible for public health insurance if they are not registered as a resident of Mexico unless they are employed by a Mexican company or have a resident visa. Private health insurance is available to all who can afford it.

> *Everything related to public healthcare is provided in Spanish only. If you don't speak Spanish, you will need an interpreter or a friend who speaks Spanish when completing paperwork or receiving treatments.*

Medical Tourism

Medical tourism is defined as going to another country to receive elective medical treatment. Each year, millions of people travel from countries that lack quality healthcare systems, to countries that provide highly-specialized medical care. In 2020, more than twenty million people traveled to other countries for medical treatments according to Patients Beyond Borders.

It makes sense that people would travel from developing nations to countries with more advanced healthcare. But a large portion of the twenty million medical tourists above are American citizens. Citizens travel to a number of different countries for reasons you will see below.

Note: This section of the guide focuses on American citizens and things that occur in the United States.

Some other countries have medical practices that meet or exceed U.S. standards, and procedures can often be done much less expensively in other countries. There are other reasons people travel outside the United States to receive medical care in addition to lower costs and higher quality. Some countries are able to provide medicine or treatments that are not available elsewhere, often due to less stringent government regulations and different cultural thinking. And sometimes it is a last resort to treat an illness like cancer that may be too aggressive or invasive for treatment in the United States.

The most common procedures medical tourists travel for are:

- cosmetic surgery,
- dental surgery,

- cardiology/heart surgery (bypass and valve replacement),
- orthopedic surgery (spinal surgery, hip and knee replacement),
- oncology (alternative cancer treatments).

Rising healthcare costs and advances in healthcare globally, have spawned a $100 billion global medical tourism industry. And countries are now in fierce competition for your business; often catering directly to American patients. Countries use the beauty and cultural aspects of their countries to combine medical procedures with the ability to be actual tourists. Countries such as Malaysia and Thailand are actively promoting medical tourism, offering medical tourism packages that include assistance with accommodations, obtaining a visa, and logistics such as airport pickups and drop-offs. Touting that medical tourists can benefit from their excellent healthcare systems and also enjoy their tourist attractions easier.

Belize for example advertises their Quality of Life Surgery Center as a leader in spinal and neurosurgical care in Central America, and entices American medical tourists with:

- top quality facilities,
- extremely well qualified & experienced surgeons,
- *only two* hours flight from Miami with your preferred airline,
- no language barrier, we are predominantly English speaking,
- monetary exchange is U.S.$1.00 to Bze$2.00,
- warm climate all year around,
- most importantly your affordable solution.

There are websites and travel agents who focus entirely on making arrangements for medical tourists. The Medical Tourism Association (MTA); a global non-profit association for the medical tourism and international patient industry, works with healthcare providers, governments, insurance companies, employers, and other buyers of healthcare—in their medical tourism, international patient, and healthcare initiatives—with a focus on providing access to transparent, high-quality healthcare (medicaltourism.com/About Us, 2021).

The Best Destinations

Not everyone agrees on the best destinations for medical tourism, but some groups create metrics which can be used as an assessment tool. Such as the Medical Tourism Index created by the Medical Tourism Association (MTA), which assesses the attractiveness of countries for medical travel, a country's economy, their public image, their healthcare costs, and their quality of care. According to the MTA, the top medical tourism destinations in 2020 were Canada, Singapore, Japan, and Spain.

Canada: Because of its close proximity to the US receives over 14 million American medical tourists each year. Canada offers quality and highly-specialized medical treatments and top-of-the-line healthcare facilities. But a spike in medical tourism recently has led to waitlists for major medical services.

Singapore: Offers excellent medical services in specialties such as oncology and cardiology. It is even leading the charge in stem cell therapy, where they are trialling the use of stem cells from bone marrow to treat diseases such as leukemia. You can save between twenty-five percent and forty percent of what you would spend on the same services in the United States. For example, heart bypass surgery costs $140,000 in the United States and $25,000 in Singapore. A hip replacement surgery which costs over $45,000 in the United States can be done for about $13,000 in Singapore.

Japan: One of the most developed healthcare systems in the world. Top-line cancer treatment centers and expertise in cosmetic surgery. Low cost is also a factor. Hip replacement surgeries that cost $30,000 in the United States are done for $4,126 in Japan. A reduction of more than seventy percent of treatment cost in the United States.

Spain: Excellent healthcare services with a beautiful travel experience. Quality healthcare services at a fraction of the cost.

Cosmetic procedures such as face lift and breast augmentation that cost as much as $15,000 in the United States cost an average of $5,000 in Spain.

(Stephano, n.d.)

Other countries such as Germany; with its advanced oncology treatments, India; known for advanced cardiac and orthopedic surgery, and South Korea; which is a world leader in spinal surgery and cancer screening, are also popular destinations.

The United States Wants a Piece of the Action

The Mayo Clinic Hospital, located in Rochester MN, was named the number one hospital in the nation, according to U.S. News & World Report's 2020-21 "Best Hospitals Honor Roll". Mayo Clinic in Rochester is the number one hospital in the nation and top ranked in twelve specialties, with number one rankings in six specialties:

- diabetes & endocrinology,
- gastroenterology (GI) & GI surgery,
- gynecology,
- nephrology,
- pulmonology & lung surgery,
- urology.

Why focus on an American hospital when millions of Americans are traveling to other countries for care? Introducing Destination Medical Center (DMC). A unique twenty-year economic development initiative which began in 2014 in Rochester MN. One of the goals of the $5.6 billion plan is to secure Mayo Clinic's and Minnesota's status as a *global* medical destination.

With the expansion of the Mayo Clinic and creation of an environment for medical innovation, education, and practice, the DMC project will effectively remake all of Rochester in the Mayo Clinic's image. Downtown will be rejuvenated and made more cold-weather friendly, while the Mayo Clinic will welcome gleaming new facilities. Vast plots of land will be used for fresh office space for biotech and pharmaceutical firms, local schools would get a cash injection, and development of amenities like hip restaurants and upscale shops will be subsidized by local and state government to attract out-of-town talent and medical tourists.

It is competing fiercely for a small-but-extremely-lucrative slice of the global medical tourism industry. Often, wealthy American and European patients have looked no further than the Mayo Clinic, but are instead choosing to get treatment abroad. But that may be changing as a result of The Destination Medical Center. (Dmc.mn, 2021)

CDC Warnings and Recommendations

The United States Centers for Disease Control (CDC) cautions that there are risks associated with medical tourism including:

- **infectious disease:** Risks associated with procedures done in other countries include wound infections, bloodstream infections, donor-derived infections, and diseases such as hepatitis B, hepatitis C, HIV.
- **antibiotic resistance:** You are more likely to get an antibiotic-resistant infection in some countries. Highly drug-resistant bacteria have caused infectious disease outbreaks among medical tourists.
- **quality of care:** Some countries' requirements for maintaining licensure, credentialing, and accreditation may also be less than what would be required in the United States. In some countries, counterfeit medicines and lower quality medical devices may be used.
- **communication challenges:** Communicating with staff at the destination and healthcare facility may be challenging. Receiving care at a facility where you do not speak the language fluently could lead to misunderstandings about your care.
- **air travel:** Flying after surgery can increase the risk for blood clots, including deep vein thrombosis.

- **continuity of care:** You may need to get healthcare in the United States if you have complications after returning.

The CDC provides the follow guidance to medical tourists:

- Medical tourists should consult with their family doctor or a travel medicine specialist for advice based on their specific health conditions, before traveling. And should also discuss any concerns they have.

- Obtain international travel health insurance that covers medical evacuation back to the United States. Your primary health insurance plan or any travel insurance you purchase will probably not cover the costs of your care while outside the country for elective procedures. And you have probably paid for your procedure or made some kind of payment arrangements before you travel. But there is the potential of additional costly expenses, you should look into how you are covered if something unexpected should occur.

- Find out what activities are not permitted after the procedure.

- Bring copies of your medical records with you Inform the medical staff at your destination of any allergies you may have.

- Pack a travel health kit with your prescription and over-the-counter medicines. Bring enough medicine to last your whole trip, plus a little extra in case of delays. Also, bring copies of all your prescriptions and a list of medications you take, including their brand names, generic names, manufacturers, and dosages.

- Get copies of all your medical records from the destination before you return home. You may need to get them translated into English.

- Check the qualifications of the healthcare providers who will be doing the procedure and the credentials of the facility where the procedure will be done.

- If you go to a country where you do not speak the language, determine ahead of time how you will communicate with your doctor and others who will be caring for you.
- Identify where you will be staying immediately after the procedure.
- Before you travel abroad for medical tourism make sure you can get any needed follow-up care in the United States.

(Centers for Disease Control and Prevention, n.d.)

Although your major medical policy or travel insurance will not cover your initial medical costs, some policies are specifically tailored for the medical tourist that will pay for the costs of complications resulting from whatever procedure you are having performed.

Accrediting groups, including Joint Commission International, DNV GL International Accreditation for Hospitals, and the International Society for Quality in Healthcare, have lists of standards that facilities need to meet to be accredited. Please note, that all surgeries carry the risk of complications, and accreditation does not guarantee a positive outcome.

Immigrants

Not all the approximately 331 million people living in the United States are U.S. citizens born in the U.S. At any given time, there are millions of immigrants living here as well accounting for five to seven percent of the population. (Immigrant simply refers to someone who was not born in the United States). There are a number of legal ways for an immigrant to be in the United States. Unfortunately, there are also around 11 million illegal or undocumented immigrants living here as well. Obviously, you do not need to be born in the United States to get sick and be in need of medical care.

Unlawfully Present / Undocumented Immigrants

According to the Kaiser Foundation, about forty-five percent of the undocumented immigrants in the US are uninsured. The remainder of them are insured through their employer, or as the spouse or dependent of an employee. Those who can afford it purchase private health insurance. They are *not* eligible to enroll in Medicare, Medicaid, or CHIP or to purchase coverage through the ACA marketplaces.

Even though they have access to private health insurance, most cannot afford it because they are working in low wage jobs (if the work at all), and since they cannot enroll in government run programs, they cannot enjoy the subsidies that are offered to everyone eligible for ACA coverage or government programs like Medicaid to help offset costs.

i

> *According to the American College of Obstetricians and Gynecologists (ACOG), some public health programs serve unauthorized immigrants, such as Title V Maternal and Child Health Services and Title X Family Planning programs. In addition, federally qualified health centers, health care for the homeless, and migrant health clinics provide comprehensive primary care, including prenatal care, without regard to income, insurance, or immigration status.* (Committee on Health Care for Underserved Women, 2015)

The burden put on the healthcare system in the United States is not analyzed in this guide. But be aware that being uninsured—as you read previously—leads to higher death rates, unpaid bills, and a number of other issues.

Lawfully Present Immigrants

The good news is, immigrants holding legal-status in the United States have access to ACA Marketplace health insurance, as well as Medicaid and Chip— with certain eligibility restrictions—and of course private health insurance. They are also eligible for all of the subsidies available through the marketplace. Still, twenty-three percent of lawfully present immigrants are uninsured due mainly to low wage jobs, or jobs that do not offer health insurance for their workers.

Immigrants with certain statuses qualify to obtain coverage on the HealthCare.gov, as well as those with applications pending for certain statuses. This is not a comprehensive list. A complete list can be obtained at: https://www.healthcare.gov/immigrants/immigration-status/

- lawful permanent resident (LPR/green card holder)
- asylee
- refugee
- individual with non-immigrant status, includes worker visas (such as H1, H-2A, H-2B), student visas, U-visa, T-visa, and other visas, and citizens of Micronesia, the Marshall Islands, and Palau
- lawful temporary resident

Source: https://www.healthcare.gov/immigrants/coverage/

Immigrants who are "qualified non-citizens" are generally eligible for coverage through Medicaid and the CHIP, if they meet their state's income and residency rules. In order to get Medicaid and CHIP coverage, many qualified non-citizens (such as many LPRs or green card holders) have a five-year waiting period. This means they must wait five years after receiving qualified immigration status before they can get

Medicaid and CHIP coverage. There are exceptions. For example, refugees, asylees, or LPRs who used to be refugees or asylees don't have to wait five years.

Source: https://www.healthcare.gov/immigrants/coverage/

Part IV – Things to Watch out For

CHAPTER 15

Common Insurance Surprises

As you navigate health insurance, many things can happen to cause you anxiety, cost you money, or even jeopardize your health. This chapter contains some common issues that occur and some helpful hints to make it easier on you along the way. Each of the items in this chapter have been introduced in previous chapters but are consolidated here as things to be aware of and cautious about.

All the solutions in the following cases should involve "ownership". You should *own* your healthcare and health insurance solutions. Be your own boss. Understand your health insurance and healthcare options and make smart educated choices about your care. Shop around, ask questions, and communicate. Don't be afraid to challenge things you are told, including charges; and if necessary, negotiate.

Don't become one of those people who wants to negotiate every charge. But if something occurs and you receive a surprise bill, it's okay to see if you can get it lowered. Make sure you understand the bill and why you have received it. Try to understand what the charges and insurance coverage are going to be *before* you get the procedure done. Communicate with your insurance company or administrator. Seek their guidance before or after a procedure to help understand charges and what has been covered and what has not. Respect healthcare professionals and the advice and medical direction they provide. But think about what they are telling you, and it's okay to challenge them too. They might not like it, but it's your health.

A lot of the things that follow do not apply during an emergency. You will have little control over what ambulance responds to your emergency, you may not have a choice of where the ambulance takes you, and you may not have a choice of what providers provide treatment. Sometimes negotiation is your only option.

<u>Surprise Bills</u>

Out-of-Network Providers

Ensure that all providers and facilities involved in your care are contracted with the network of your health insurance plan. Don't make assumptions; actually ask. You should always ask what providers will be performing billable services when having inpatient or outpatient surgery and if they are in-network. For example, your in-network provider may sometimes use labs or other third parties during your treatment that are not in your network. If the services you are having performed are not available from a contracted provider or if you can't wait to make arrangements or will have to travel a great distance, contact your insurance company or administrator and discuss alternatives with them.

If a provider refers you elsewhere for services, always verify that the provider or facility you are being referred to is in your network. Asking your original provider or his staff is okay, but you should verify with your insurer to be sure, since your doctor and his office staff may not be aware of all other providers' network status, and they surely do not know the details of your health insurance plan.

If your provider or facility has been in-network, don't assume they are in-network on *this* visit. Ask the office staff to confirm.

Many plans contain provisions for using out-of-network providers or facilities in extreme circumstances such as a particular provider type being more than thirty-five miles away. If you do plan to utilize an out-of-network provider, coordinate with them in advance to determine what they will accept as payment. Understand how your insurance treats out-of-network providers and how they determine the allowable. You might have a real need or desire to go out-of-network. Understand that it is going to cost you more, but do your homework so you minimize the cost and are not surprised. If you have concerns, always discuss them with your insurance company.

Providers You Didn't Know Were Part of Your Treatment

Your provider is in-network, the hospital you have chosen is in-network, and you still have received large bills from the surgical assistant, the anesthesiologist, the nurse, and the lab that performed your blood work. Depending on what service you are having performed, there could be numerous people in addition to your physician who are involved. That is a drastic case. Most networks have good participation. But there is no guarantee that every one of those providers is in your network just because the hospital is in-network.

When having a procedure performed, you need to ask whether everybody involved in your care is an in-network provider. If not, you should ask if there are other options.

As mentioned in earlier chapters, many states are now passing laws against these kinds of surprise bills, and it is also part of many political candidates' platforms. Since self-insured plans are not governed by state laws, they may not need to abide by state laws that are passed regarding surprise medical bills. Many health insurance plans have provisions built in regarding this situation, so be sure to check your plan, or call your insurer.

i

> *Something people are not aware of or forget is that the facility where you have a treatment done may charge you for the use of their facility. in or outpatient surgeries are performed in operating rooms that are often not owned by the provider, and charge separately for their use.*

Preventive Care / Well Visits

Routine visits **for preventive services** are covered at no cost to you when you see a doctor in your network. Office visits when you are not sick, referred to as "well visits", must be covered one hundred percent (you may need to pay a small copay) under the provisions of the Affordable Care Act. Many services—such as routine physical exams, vaccinations, and even routine screening colonoscopies—must be covered by the insurer at no cost to the insured.

However, if the scope of your visit increases, you *may* be charged. An increase in scope could be something as minor as a discussion with your doctor about a past or current condition. Don't be afraid to ask how something will be billed. If your plan is grandfathered, essential health benefits are not required to be done with no charge. Although grandfathered plans are becoming scarce.

Also, be aware that a screening colonoscopy is different from a diagnostic colonoscopy. **A screening or preventative colonoscopy is** performed on a person without symptoms for the purpose of testing for the presence of colorectal cancer or colorectal polyps. It does not matter if polyps or cancer is found. The intent of the original screening does not change. A diagnostic procedure is performed on a patient who has gastrointestinal symptoms or who has past or present polyps or gastrointestinal disease. A diagnostic colonoscopy is not required to be covered by insurance.

i

> *Although a screening colonoscopy is covered at one hundred percent per ACA rules, if the doctor removes a polyp and sends it to a lab for analysis, the lab work is NOT covered at one hundred percent; however, it does not change the fact that the original procedure was preventative.*

Emergency Room Visits

Your emergency room benefit covers treatments you receive in the emergency room when you are released the same day. If you go to the emergency room but are taken to another part of the hospital for observation, surgery, or reasons other than diagnostic testing, it is usually considered an admission, which is treated differently from an emergency room visit.

After an emergency hospital admission, you or a responsible party usually has a certain number of days to notify your insurance company or administrator. Otherwise, your benefits may be reduced. The hospital will normally notify the insurance company for you but not always. You should always ask the facility if they have notified your insurance company (if you are able). Another issue with emergency rooms is that they sometimes use contractors instead of hospital doctors. The contractors may or may not be part of your health insurance plan's network.

Preauthorization

You need to be aware of what services require preauthorization under your plan, and verify that it has occurred. Most doctors know how and when to do this, but be sure to verify. Or do the notification yourself. If a service requires preauthorization and you fail to obtain it, then your benefits could be significantly reduced, or there may be no benefit at all.

Occurrences

Know that there may be limits on certain benefits in your plan and understand what they are. Plans have limits on the number of times you can receive a particular treatment, lab, or diagnostic test in a specific period. A common limit on dental plans is that fillings are allowed only once on the same tooth every eighteen months, and panoramic X-rays are allowed only once every three years. Another example is physical therapy. Your plan may only cover a certain number of visits.

Covered Services

Your provider may tell you a service is covered by your health insurance plan, but it's up to you to know or verify. Your providers and their staff cannot know all the details of your health insurance plan. There may be certain tests that are specifically excluded under your plan or there may be restrictions on what kinds of facilities you may visit. Some health insurance plans only pay for X-rays and other diagnostic testing that is done in a free-standing facility as opposed to a hospital (which is normally much more expensive). Also, some procedures may have only partial coverage.

Discuss all your treatment with your providers and, if necessary, with your insurance company or administrator. There may be alternative tests that fall within your coverage that will be less expensive. If your plan will only pay a portion of a covered service or a maximum amount, you may be able to use cost transparency tools and other means to shop around to find a less expensive provider.

Pre-existing conditions

A pre-existing condition is an illness or injury that you have before you start a new health care plan. Conditions like diabetes, COPD, cancer, and sleep apnea, are examples of what could be considered a pre-existing health condition. Pre-existing conditions tend to be chronic or long-term, and usually one for which you have received treatment or diagnosis before you enrolled in a new health plan. Prior to 2010 and the passage of the Affordable Care Act (ACA), you could be denied coverage or charged inflated prices if it was determined you had a pre-existing condition. The ACA made it illegal for health insurance companies to deny you medical coverage or raise rates due to a pre-existing condition.

If, however, you are enrolled in one of those grandfathered health insurance plans, (a plan that started before 2010) these plans can cancel your coverage or charge you higher rates due to a pre-existing condition, but that would probably have been done already.

The ACA says they cannot deny you coverage or charge you higher rates, but the benefits related to your pre-existing condition may not be the same. Some private health insurance plans put a dollar limit on how much they will pay if you have a medical problem related to a specific pre-existing condition.

Ambulances

Most ambulance services used to be free of charge. They have been provided by volunteers or town fire departments. Today ambulances are highly privatized and usually charge by the mile, as well as other charges for materials they use. The companies that run the ambulances and the insurance companies cannot agree on what is a fair price, so the ambulance companies do not join networks. An ambulance ride could cost several hundred if not thousands of dollars, with a large portion of that being patient responsibility.

Ambulance insurance is often available through the ambulance company, the city, or a third-party insurer as an add-on policy. This can be a very economical option that could potentially save you from a large unexpected bill.

Even more concerning are air ambulances that transfer critically ill patients who need to get to a specific trauma center very quickly. An air ambulance ride could cost as much as $25,000. Very little of this charge is usually covered by insurance, and in many cases air ambulances are specifically excluded from plans because of the potential cost.

Examples

In most of the examples below, issues may have been avoided with better communication. Assuming your insurer would provide accurate information and guide you through diagnosis and treatment plans, they will let you know what is covered and what is not, potentially giving you choices and empowering you in your care.

Surprise Medical Bills Totaling $18,000

Early one morning, a man woke with severed stomach pain. He was taken to the emergency room of a local hospital. He specifically asked to be taken to *that* hospital because it was in-network. An X-ray showed an enlarged gallbladder and surgery was performed to removed it.

A few months later, he received a bill from the surgeon for $18,000. After discussion with his insurer, it was discovered that the surgeon they called to perform the gallbladder surgery was out-of-network and he brought in another colleague to assist who was also out-of-network.

His insurer paid the first surgeon after negotiating a reduced rate. But they refused to pay the second surgeon's bill. The patient spoke with the hospital and was told that they call in whichever emergency doctor is on-call at that time and there was nothing they could do about his bill or the insurers unwillingness to pay.

Unable to pay the bill, it was turned over to collections. (Wong, 2019)

Surprise Medical Bills Totaling $19,000

A family was out for a bicycle ride when their young son crashed. They called 911 because he required stitches. An ambulance took him to the Emergency Room for treatment, and after some stitches he was fine.

A few weeks later the family received a bill from the hospital for nearly $19,000. The EOB they received from their insurer said, their claim had been denied and their patient responsibility would be the entire sum of $18,933.44. Because the coding on the claim indicated that the injuries were the result of an accident, the insurer felt that financial responsibility should fall with someone else. They did not know *who,* but there was an investigation in progress.

In this case, the father was an attorney which helped him understand his options. He did what everyone should do - he asked questions, and he fought until the insurer did what they should have done in the first place. They paid $7,414.76 of the cost. The family owed only $1,853.45, which represented their share of the deductible and copay. (Julie Appleby; KHN, 2020)

Surprise Medical Bills Totaling $28,000

A 28-year-old man experienced severe stomach pain and a high fever, and was rushed to the closest emergency room which happened to be an out-of-network hospital. They performed several tests, and determined that he had appendicitis, for which they performed emergency surgery that night. He was released and went home the next day.

A few weeks later, the man received a bill from the hospital for $28,295. The total bill was $42,212 for surgery, one night at the hospital and the emergency room charges. He received an EOB from his insurer that said they paid $8,944. His responsibility consisted of his $4,000 deductible and coinsurance, and the remainder of the $41,212 in charges.

He was "balance billed" because he went to an out-of-network hospital — and even though it was an emergency, the insurer did not see it that way. He went to court to challenge the bill because the charge was so far out of line with the $6,000 - $13,000 considered to be a fair and reasonable price for the laparoscopic appendectomy in his area, according to Healthcare Bluebook. (Julie Appleby; KHN, 2020)

Surprise Medical Bills Totaling $40,000

After a long illness and lots of medical tests, a woman was diagnosed with sarcoma; a type of cancer that begins in bone or in the soft tissues of the body. She began chemotherapy treatment immediately.

She began receiving claim denials and bills from providers for some of the tests that were conducted, so she contacted her insurer to find out what was going on. She was informed that many of the diagnostic tests were not going to be covered, either because they were deemed unnecessary or experimental.

Her insurance is covering the cost of the chemotherapy treatments, but it appears that she is responsible for close to $40,000.

She has begun appeals of denied claims. She is out of work due to her illness, taking care of her children, and generally feeling too sick to get out of bed some days because of the chemotherapy. Now she has the prospect of large medical debt adding to her stress and contributing to the decline of her overall health. (Wong, 2019)

Surprise Medical Bills Totaling $64,000

A woman was diagnosed with Severe Crohn's disease. She was prescribed an oral medication but after several weeks, it was obvious that she needed more aggressive treatment. She was prescribed infusion therapy with Remicade. Because of the cost of this treatment, the doctor and the woman both contacted her insurance to get the procedure pre-authorized. After some back-and-forth, the insurer agreed that the therapy was medically necessary.

She felt good about complying with the precertification requirements of her plan and she began the treatment. After a few weeks, she received an EOB that said her claim was denied because the treatment was not covered as part of her health insurance plan's benefits. She soon received a bill for $21,000 for one infusion. At that point, she had already had three infusions. Assuming the same thing was going to happen with the other two infusions, she contacted her insurer. The insurer's response was, "Just because we approved the medicine, doesn't mean it's covered." She received bills for a total of $64,000. (Wong, 2019)

Surprise Medical Bills Totaling Over $100,000

A woman and her husband flew to California to visit relatives. While in California they were involved in a serious car accident, which results in serious injuries to the woman. She of course was taken to the hospital for emergency treatment which included examinations, x-rays, inpatient care, and medications. However, that hospital was unable to provide the care she needed, they were offered a choice to fly to Las Vegas or Salt Lake City for further tests and treatment. It would have been a four-hour drive via ground ambulance.

She was flown to Salt Lake City where she received the treatment she needed. She remembers someone coming to her room to explain her insurance, but was heavily sedated and cannot recall the details of the conversation.

When they returned home, they received a bill for $60,000. The insurer decided that the plane ride was elective, and they should have chosen the ground ambulance.

They appealed four times, and the ER doctor documented that the Air Ambulance was medically necessary and they were not given an option of a ground ambulance. While the appeals were happening, the bill gathered interest and grew to $75,000 for just the air ambulance. The total debt was close to $100,000.

All four appeals were denied, and they declared bankruptcy.(Sultan, 2020)

Summary

Before getting a medical procedure or tests, understand how much of it will be covered by your health insurance plan. The first step is making sure a doctor has approved or requested the necessary treatment or tests. Even though your doctor ordered a test, it does not mean the insurer will consider it medically necessary (see preauthorization), and that may be a requirement of your plan.

Read your health insurance documents, or call your health insurance provider and ask them what kind of coverage you have for a specific procedure or test. Some insurance companies have websites with covered procedures listed, but your most accurate information will come from the documents that specifically describe your plan or policy. Also, understand that there may be exclusions or limitations for the amount the insurer will reimburse.

Look for limits on how many times you will be covered for a specific service, test, or treatment such as X-rays or other scans. Sometimes a health insurance plan will limit the number of times, or the total amount payable for a procedure. Finding out if it's covered may not tell the entire story. Be cognizant of the networks that providers belong to and try to find out what other providers, labs and the like may be part of your care (will bill you). Be familiar with the network affiliation of the closest Emergency Room, and where the closest hospital that is in your health insurance plan's network for you is located.

Obtain a predetermination of benefits or pretreatment estimate. This is a formal inquiry of your coverage. A predetermination typically includes your eligibility status, covered services, amounts payable, copayments, deductibles, and plan maximums.

Use cost transparency tools or whatever methods you have to try to determine how much a procedure will cost, and shop around for the best price. It is not wise to always try to find the cheapest doctor you can find. Your health is not something you want to go cheap on. Also read reviews and pay attention to quality indicators for providers and factor them into your decisions. But with the range of prices among equally competent providers for identical services, price shopping is a smart thing to do.

If you get a bill from a provider and you are not going to be able to pay it right away, call the provider and try to arrange either a payment plan or an extension. If you just ignore it, it will likely be sent to a collection agency and show up on your credit report as unpaid. Providers will often work with you.

Lastly, talk to your insurance company or administrator. They will be glad to talk to you and discuss what your insurance will cover and how it will be applied. If you have been able to obtain costs from the provider, you will even be able to get your insurer to estimate the portion of the charges that you will be responsible for paying.

Part V – Advanced Topics

CHAPTER 16

Controlling Healthcare
Costs and Quality

Transparency

We live in a free-market society. We have price competition, which is one of the ways products and services compete in the marketplace. For two products that are similar in function and quality, cost is the next differentiator.

Gasoline stations on opposite sides of the street compete based on price. As one lowers the price a penny, the other follows suit so they do not lose customers. When one raises the price a few cents, the other can do the same without losing customers. They have large signs advertising the price of their gasoline. But what if the price of gasoline is secret? What if you couldn't compare prices? What if you do not know the price you are paying for gasoline until *after* you fill your tank? There's little incentive to keep the prices low if you are not going to tell anyone how much gasoline costs. That is exactly what occurs in healthcare most of the time. It is part of the reason people often say that the system is broken, and one of the things people point to when discussing why Healthcare costs are high. It is detrimental not only to consumers but also to providers, facilities, and insurers.

In a report from the American College of Physicians (ACP), the Institute of Medicine (IOM) defines healthcare transparency as "making available to the public, in a reliable, and understandable manner, information on the healthcare system's quality, efficiency and consumer experience with care, which includes price and quality data, so as to influence the behavior of patients, providers, payers, and others to achieve better outcomes (quality and cost of care)".

Price transparency includes:

- physicians, hospitals and other providers publicizing their usual charges for particular healthcare services;

- insurers making available to their subscribers the rates that they have negotiated with physicians and hospitals;

- government agencies publicly reporting the average prices for common healthcare services.

Source: (ACPOnline.org, 2010)

Your healthcare and health insurance experience will be higher quality and less expensive if you understand the cost of medical services before they are performed and better for everyone because it will help keep costs in check.

On November 15, 2019 Pres. Donald Trump issued an executive order to Improve Price and Quality Transparency in American Healthcare. The goal of the executive order is to help consumers know the price and quality of a good or service and to make informed decisions about their health care. Other rules have also recently been issued for drug manufacturers to disclose list prices in their advertisements and require hospitals to publish list prices on their websites. The executive order is not itself a change in law or regulations. Rather, it is a directive to government agencies to draft new rules or guidance. (Keith, 2019)

According to the Centers for Medicare & Medicaid Services, starting January 1, 2021, all hospitals operating in the United States will be required to

provide clear, accessible pricing information online about the items and services they provide in two ways:

- as a comprehensive machine-readable file with all items and services.
- in a display of shoppable services in a consumer-friendly format.

Hospital price transparency helps Americans know the cost of a hospital item or service before receiving it, and will make it easier for consumers to shop and compare prices across hospitals and estimate the cost of care before going to the hospital.

Tools exist that consumers can use to help determine costs for medical services from different providers, and shop around for low-cost providers. These tools currently exist, and are quickly gaining popularity among employers, insurers and consumers. Cost transparency not only allows the consumer to better understand costs but also results in cost savings to the employee and employer. A cost transparency tool could be very helpful for someone with a high deductible health plan who is trying to manage costs, by comparing cost and quality to stay within the funds in an HSA.

Let's say your employer is self-insured, and you need an x-ray. Let's even say that you have met your deductible so the service will be covered with twenty percent coinsurance. You use one of the cost transparency tools, and you discover that instead of going to a giant corporate hospital and getting charged five-hundred dollars, you can go to the free-standing radiology clinic down the street and be charged two-hundred dollars for the same X-ray. So instead of the employer and employee paying $400 and $100 respectively, the employer and employee pay $160 and $40 respectively. That is a realistic example.

An example is, a colonoscopy with biopsy in one particular city has a price range of $1,200 to $3,800. That's a difference of over two hundred percent. The tool also informs you that $2,154 is a fair price for this medical procedure. So you can see that the range of prices for medical services can be extreme.

Transparency is not just about costs. It is also about the quality of service you receive. Some of these tools also contain reviews of the providers, and sometimes they contain quality indicators as well. If you have your choice, you'll pick a five-star hotel over a three-star hotel if the price is similar. The same should go for your healthcare providers.

Some companies that provide transparency tools also offer a rewards program. In the example above, the employer may be willing to reward the employee with $50 since they have chosen a provider that has saved them $240. The rewards will vary based on the savings to the employer. But any way you look at it, everyone benefits from cost transparency.

The companies that provide this service usually charge a fee for using them. One or more of them is often included in your insurance plan, but not always. If not, you should ask your employer, especially if your employer is self-insured. These tools have documented positive results.

Reference-Based Pricing

Another cost-savings tool that is gaining momentum lately is called reference-based pricing (RBP). RBP is not a tool that the consumer uses like the tools described above. Instead, this tool is used by the insurer to determine allowable charges similar to in-network pricing which was discussed earlier. Many employer-sponsored health insurance plans are turning to RBP to help lower their healthcare-related costs. With charges varying so much between providers, this tool helps insurers to standardize pricing and instead of an allowable charge based on a network discount, the allowable charges are based on what is considered fair and reasonable.

How is the "reasonable" amount determined? Before discussing that, we need to first explore healthcare pricing in general. When we discussed provider networks, we said that the providers who are members of a network, agree to accept a discounted fee for their services when you have health insurance plans that contract with the same provider network of the provider. The fact is that the amount providers charge for their services is overinflated to account for the discounts that they are going to give to a majority of their patients.

Out-of-network providers can charge more because they are not forced to accept any discounts and they can charge whatever they want because you do not have the transparency to compare with other providers. The difference in charges for the same service from one provider to the next is wide as seen in the previous discussion on transparency. According to Kaiser Health News, out-of-network providers charge patients on average three hundred percent more than the Medicare rate for certain treatments or procedures. Studies have found that some treatments are even more exorbitant — with out-of-network providers charging nearly 1,400 percent more than what is reimbursed by Medicare. (Gorman, 2015)

Healthgram, a health plan administrator cites the following example to illustrate the disparity in charges. "The average charge for a major joint replacement at a hospital in North Carolina is $59,622. Typical big insurance discounts will slash that price by fifty percent to around $30,000. The discounted price seems fair until you compare it to the Medicare price of $9,264. Medicare often reimburses at cost, leaving no margin for the facility and providers" (Healthgram.com, 2020).

What if there is a way to cut through all the discounts, and over-inflated charges and figure out what is actually a fair (reasonable) price? Additionally, what if you could get providers to accept this "fair" price? That's where reference-based pricing comes in. In this model, the amount that the health insurance plan will pay, is based on the actual cost to the provider of the service(s), and then a fair and reasonable amount is added on top for provider profit. There is no consideration of in or out-of-network, or the actual provider charges. The resulting rate usually ends up being 120 to three hundred percent of the Medicare rates, which is what a Medicare participating provider is required to accept for the same service(s).

Similar to the model for an out-of-network provider, the provider sends in a claim, and the administrator says, "Here's a fair amount we are willing to pay." But in this case, the provider is expected to accept the amount offered. In fact, insurers require that the provider accepts the amount they will pay. There is no guarantee that the provider will accept the price, and they may balance bill you because there is no network contract binding them.

Insurers team with entities who specialize in RBP litigation and negotiation. If your health insurance plan utilizes RBP, you will be told that there will not be or should not be any balance billing, and if you receive a bill from the provider, you should notify the RBP entity and they will handle it.

There have been lawsuits filed by providers over balance billing issues, but most have been settled out of court. "Most often, the provider ends up accepting the RBP amount as payment in full before things reach that stage. In those instances where providers won't accept the RBP rate, the plan will negotiate a settlement or pay the outstanding bill" (Hroncich, A how-to guide for reference-based pricing, 2019). Many facilities and other providers are aware of this method of pricing, and as it gains popularity, they are opting to accept RBP instead of spending the time and effort to fight it, and to ensure that patients are not steered away from them.

Quality of Care

The healthcare payment model that has been discussed so far in this guide is called "fee-for-service", which means the provider charges a fee for each service which is then paid by you or the insurance company. In this model, provider revenues are driven by volume. The more patients a provider sees, the more revenue the practice receives. There is no incentive for the provider to provide quality care (other than their Hippocratic oath). There's a saying (although no provider would admit to saying it) that goes, "A sick patient is worth more than a healthy patient".

As healthcare costs continue to rise, providers and insurers are exploring alternative payment models (APM) that are focused on value rather than volume. In other words, they are searching for ways to improve quality of care while keeping costs down. It may seem odd that the part of this guide called "quality of care" is focused on how provider's charge for their services. But as you will see in the following sections, they are directly related.

Bundled Pricing

One alternative payment model is called "bundled pricing". In this pricing model, instead of paying for each service individually, the cost is bundled into a single fee for an "episode of care". It is not intended for an office visit, lab test, or minor services. It is geared toward an "event" or "episode" where multiple providers and multiple visits are involved, such as heart surgery, joint replacement surgery, or labor and delivery of a child. Since it usually involves multiple visits, it is usually priced as a cost for a period. For example, a knee replacement bundle might be $15,000 over thirty days, and then you are entitled to several visits before and after the surgery as well as the surgery itself for that price.

Bundled pricing incentivizes providers to move toward better coordination, efficiency, and quality of care by having the provider(s) assume the risk. With bundled pricing, the total costs of all services you receive for a particular episode are estimated based on historical claims over a period, factoring in pre-operative visits, post-operative visits, and therapies. Then the bundled price is the allowable fee paid by the insurance company. The provider assumes the risk because if the cost of treatment, including treatment of complications and hospital re-admissions, is more than what has been estimated, the providers are responsible. If, however, through collaboration and efficiency the providers are able to keep the cost down and provide a service with a quality outcome for less than the reimbursed bundled amount, then the providers share in the savings.

Insurers, employers, and employees all like this kind of APM because they benefit from the savings created by quality outcomes in addition to the providers. According to a study in the *Journal of the American Medical Association (JAMA)* published in 2017, "In this observational study of 3942 patients who received joint replacement surgery, there was a decrease of $5577 (20.8 percent) in total spending per episode" (Amol S. Navathe, 2017). The study was performed at Baptist Health Systems, a recognized leader in healthcare in San Antonio and South Texas, from July 2008 to June 2015. Hospital systems across the country have been experimenting with APMs and variations of bundled payment reimbursement. CMS has also been experimenting with bundled payments for certain kinds of surgeries (mainly joint replacement) for several years to reduce costs and improve quality of care.

Direct Primary Care (DPC) and Concierge Medicine

The term APM is a health insurance industry term. DPC is not technically an APM because one of the reasons DPC arrangements are attractive is that they bypass health insurance altogether.

In the late 1990s, a group of doctors and investors in Seattle, Washington had a plan to revolutionize the healthcare industry with a business model for primary care physicians called direct primary care. In this business model, you pay a monthly fee directly to a doctor, and then you have exclusive access to that provider for routine office visits, simple testing, and coordination of care. None of the services get billed to a third-party insurer, which is why it is referred to as "direct" care.

There is currently a healthcare problem in the United States that affects family physicians, pediatricians, and OB/GYNs. As you will read throughout this guide, the insurance companies and networks almost completely dictate what these providers are paid for their services. Providers need to be members of networks to compete, and with lower and lower payments from insurance, they are forced to see as many patients as possible to maintain a profitable revenue stream. This shifts the focus from quality to quantity.

With the DPC model, you pay a monthly fee directly to a provider (like a membership fee), which is usually less than $100. There are then no charges for office visits and simple tests, no deductibles, and no coinsurance or copays, and you generally receive better, more personal care. Physicians like the model because it allows them to limit the number of patients they see, which then allows them to spend more time with each patient; and with less administrative tasks associated with insurance, it allows their practices to spend more time on the practice of medicine. If you need to go to a specialist, or need treatment beyond what can be provided by a family practice, you will need to either have supplemental insurance or pay out-of-pocket. But physicians who have DPC practices are sometimes able to negotiate discounts with local labs, specialists, and hospitals.

According to an article in the University of Pennsylvania's Wharton School of Business magazine in 2019, "[T]here are approximately 465,000 physicians in the U.S. who practice primary care (internists, family physicians, pediatric, and OB/GYN). Of these primary care physicians, approximately 20,000 physicians (mainly internal and family medicine) practice some sort of DPC. This constitutes approximately 4.5 percent of the entire primary care workforce. The number of physicians practicing DPC has grown at a fairly rapid pace over the past five years or so" (Voigt, 2019). Since it has only existed for a short time, there is little data available. But most physicians have reported that it has resulted in increased revenue while providing a higher quality of care for their patients.

Concierge medicine is similar to DPC, or is a type of DPC. In this model, physicians are usually still part of a network and still bill insurance. You will still pay a fee, which is usually a yearly membership and the fee is higher than a DPC fee. But you will get such perks as "24/7 access, a cell phone number to connect directly with their physician, same-day appointments, visits that last as long as it takes to address their needs and varying other amenities. In exchange for this enhanced access and personal attention, the Concierge Doctor receives a fee, which enables them to increase the amount of time they spend with Patients" (What is Concierge Medicine? [Updated for 2020], 2020). If you are able to pay a little more than others for your healthcare, you can receive preferential treatment by subscribing with a concierge doctor. This is popular with celebrities and other high-profile people.

CHAPTER 17

Where Does the
Money Come From?

Does it seem to you like insurance companies are big money trees, and when you need them to pay for something, you just shake the tree and they pay the medical bills? It might seem like that, but that's not exactly how it works. But if the money does not grow on trees, then where does it come from?

A portion of the money that an insurance company uses to pay your medical expenses comes from the insurance premiums they collect from you. Depending on what kind of plan you have and whether you have private insurance or an employer-sponsored plan, where the remainder of the money comes from varies. This chapter will explain where the money comes from and how insurers are protected against very large claims.

Medicare

For the Medicare program described in a previous chapter, claims are paid by the federal government from the Medicare trust. The trust is funded by a combination of payroll taxes, premiums of those on Medicare and funding from the federal government. Medicare funding is a line-item in the federal budget that is often either cut or increased depending on other areas of need and the political affiliation of the president and Congress. The total Medicare payments for 2018 totaled over $389 billion for Parts A and B (CMS.gov, 2018) and over $168 billion for Part D (CMS.gov, 2018).

For non-Medicare health insurance plans, there are two different kinds of claim funding arrangements, fully-insured and self-insured.

Fully-Insured

Under a fully-insured arrangement, an insurance company (like Blue Cross, Cigna, and Aetna) assumes all the responsibility of paying your claims *and* most of the risk that goes along with it. Just like auto insurance, or homeowner's insurance, they collect premiums from those they insure, pay claims within the rules of the plan, and count on a portion of the insured members having no or a small number of claims and offset those with claims they have to pay. The money to pay claims comes completely from premiums you and others pay for the insurance.

The insurance companies spend a great deal of effort to determine what your premium should be based on several factors including your claims they have paid previously. Factors that are taken into account when determining premium rates that are competitive to the consumer and profitable to the company are described below. Since the insurance company assumes most of the risk, and the money they pay out comes entirely from premiums from the insured members, the premiums for this type of insurance are higher. Your rates may increase when the company incurs a large number of claims in the previous year even if they are not your claims.

The year after Hurricane Katrina devastated parts of Louisiana, auto insurance rates for some insurance companies increased significantly because they had a large proportion of their insured members in that region of the country. They incurred large losses beyond what they collected in premiums, in the previous year because of the massive hurricane. They were forced to charge everyone they insured more money to make up for the losses in the previous year. That example is not health insurance related, but it applies equally to health insurance, and illustrates how rates are affected from year-to-year based on how much the insurer paid out the previous year.

Self-Insured

There is another option called "self-insurance". In this arrangement, your employer sponsors a health insurance plan for you and your coworkers, and assumes most of the risk. The employer (the insurer) itself collects a premium from you (their employees) and they are responsible for paying all claims. For this reason, these types of insurance plans are also referred to as "self-funded". A third-party administrator is almost always involved to handle all the administrative tasks associated with paying claims, as well as providing other health-insurance-related services.

The TPA works with the employer and brokers to determine the premiums for the employees based (as with fully insured) on the previous claims paid by the employees of the company (assuming the employer has provided health insurance previously) and the concept of those without claims paying for those with claims. Because the employer assumes most of the risk, the premiums that you pay can be lower. The employer pays for the services provided by the TPA, and for claims from premiums collected, supplemented by funds from the business. They can adjust the amount that they ask you to pay for premiums by contributing more or less of their own money.

In a 2019 report to Congress, the Department of Labor said, "In 2016, self-insured plans covered forty-six percent of plan participants, mixed-funded plans thirty-seven percent, and fully insured plans eighteen percent. (Percentages do not sum to one hundred percent because of rounding)" (Constantijn W.A. Panis PhD; Michael J. Brien PhD, 2019). Mixed-funded plans are employers who offer their employees fully-insured and self-insured plan options.

Large companies are more likely to self-insure because they have more financial resources available. However, more and more small companies are now self-insuring because it saves them money. A Kaiser Health News report says that "[a]mong companies with 5,000 or more employees, ninety-four percent of covered workers were in self-funded plans" (Bazar, For Millions of Insured Americans, State Health Laws Don't Apply, 2017).

For people in self-funded plans, most state healthcare laws do not apply. However, self-insured group health plans come under all applicable federal laws, including the Employee Retirement Income Security Act (ERISA).

According to the Self-Insurance Institute of America (SIIA), there are several reasons why employers choose the self-insurance option.

- The employer can customize the plan to meet the specific healthcare needs of its workforce. Not forced to accept a one-size-fits-all policy
- The employer maintains control over the money. This maximum interest income.
- The employer does not have to pre-pay for coverage, creating improved cash flow.
- The employer is not subject to conflicting state health insurance regulations/benefit mandates as self-insured health plans are regulated under federal law (ERISA).
- The employer is not subject to state health insurance premium taxes, which are usually two to three percent of the premiums.
- The employer is free to contract with the providers or provider network best suited to meet the healthcare needs of its employees

Source: (SIIA, 2019)

The first reason in the list above talks about flexibility. With a fully-insured health insurance plan, the insurance company may offer a few benefit options, but you are forced to choose from the options they offer. Since they are assuming all the risk, they are very careful about deviating from the benefits they offer.

A self-insured plan, on the other hand, has limitless possibilities for benefit offerings. This is where a broker comes in handy. A broker is an insurance expert who collects a fee and acts as a consultant for an employer to help them build benefit plans to provide their employees. Together, the broker, an administrator, and the employer build benefit plans for the employer to offer their employees as cost-effectively as possible. Brokers work closely with employers and TPAs throughout the process and continue to provide consultation to the employer during the benefit year.

Unfortunately, since state insurance regulation does not apply to self-insured plans, they also do not get to enjoy any of the protections offered by state regulation. One example is that they do not get to take advantage of laws that many states have adopted pertaining to surprise medical bills. The good news is that employers usually have the best interest of their employers in mind and design things into their plans to counter any of the issues created by self-funding. For instance, one of the common reasons for surprise medical bills is out-of-network anesthesiologists. Most self-insured plans have provisions to treat them as in-network if they are not already.

In a self-funded arrangement, the employer is responsible for paying the claims, so they need to have sufficient financial resources (cash flow). You cannot predict with one hundred percent certainty how many claims your employees are going to have and for how much. But in this arrangement, the employer has complete control over the funds used to pay claims.

Premiums

If you attempt to obtain individual private health insurance, the insurer is not allowed to use your prior health history in determining your premium rate. The Affordable Care Act contains rules about how an insurance company can determine your premium. By law, they can only account for the following five things:

- Age: Older people pay higher premiums
- Geographic location.
- Tobacco use: Smokers will pay higher premiums
- Individual versus family enrollment: The premium will be higher if it covers more people.
- Benefits: The actual benefits provided in the plan, and how cost-sharing is structured (how much the insurer pays versus how much the insured pays).

By law, they cannot take your gender, or your current health, or medical history into account.

For employer-sponsored group health insurance plans, the claims paid for the employees have a much greater impact on the premiums because there are less people to spread the expenses across. GMS, a national TPA and consulting firm, lists the following items that group health insurance plans can take into account when determining premiums:

- Size of the group: A larger group of people can help lower your premium by spreading the associated health risks over an entire group.

- Health of the group: The Affordable Care Act doesn't allow insurers to change premiums or deny insurance based on an individual's pre-existing conditions. However, for group plans, the overall health of the group can play a role in determining premiums.

- Average age of your group: The Affordable Care Act allows insurers to consider age of the group in premium determinations.

- An employer's collective claims history: Insurance providers use the number of total claims and how expensive those claims are to determine your premiums.

- Type of occupation: Different lines of work carry different levels of risk.

- Benefits: As with individual private insurance, the actual benefits provided in the plan, and how cost-sharing is structured play a significant role in determining premium.

Source: (Austin, 2017)

Reinsurance / Stop Loss

Have you noticed in the section above on self-insured versus fully-insured plans that either the insurance company or the employer assumes *most* of the risk? This is because, in the self-insured world, any employer who takes on the responsibility of funding health insurance claims most likely purchases insurance to transfer some of the risk to other parties. Those other parties are called reinsurers.

If a small self-insured business has an employee who gets a critical illness and has $500,000 in claims, it could wipe out the business financially. Because they are self-insured, they are responsible financially for all claims for their employees. But, by purchasing reinsurance (sometimes called stop-loss), they can be assured that they will not need to pay over a certain amount.

One type of reinsurance will assume the risk of any single claim being greater than some dollar amount. For instance, $100,000 maybe the limit placed on a single claim. Another type of reinsurance assumes the risk that the total dollar amount of a single person's claims, or the entire employer's claims will not go over a certain dollar threshold;

maybe $250,000. The higher these limits are, the lower the reinsurance premium will be.

Reinsurance is not exclusive to health insurance. Insurance is a type of risk management for any entity who is at risk of loss of any kind. Mostly every person, business, or organization has some kind of insurance protecting them from some kind of loss. And anyone who is a reinsurer, is also at a risk of loss if they have too many claims, so they will also transfer some of the risk to other reinsurers. In our economy, any huge losses are rarely assumed by any single party. And it is why when a natural disaster occurs, the risk as well as the loss is spread out over many different insurers and re-insurers.

CHAPTER 18

Health Insurance Fraud

In this chapter, you will learn about insurance fraud and see some of the penalties that have been imposed on people who have been caught committing this crime.

Insurance companies and administrators are always on the lookout for fraud and other dishonest activity. They do this by scrutinizing all claims they receive in various ways. Sometimes, a provider may try to collect more money from the insurer than they are entitled to. When a provider submits claims for fictitious people, or pads a claim with services that have not been provided, it is considered insurance fraud, which has stiff penalties.

The Health Insurance Portability and Accountability Act of 1996 officially established healthcare fraud as a federal crime. Penalties could be a federal prison term of up to ten years in addition to significant fines and restitution. The FBI is the primary investigative agency involved in the fight against healthcare insurance fraud, and Medicare Fraud is by-far where the majority of the fraud occurs. According to the Department of Justice website, in fiscal year 2019, the fraud task force accomplishments included:

- Filing 359 indictments and complaints involving charges filed against 673 defendants who allegedly billed federal health care programs more than $5.1 billion
- Obtaining 323 guilty pleas negotiated and 33 jury trials litigated, with guilty verdicts against 35 defendants
- Securing imprisonment for 340 defendants sentenced, averaging nearly 49 months of incarceration

Source: (USDOJ, Retrieved 4/21/21)

Ten common healthcare provider fraud schemes according to the Association of Certified Fraud Examiners (ACFE), are,

- billing for services not rendered,
- billing for a non-covered service as a covered service,
- misrepresenting dates of service,
- misrepresenting locations of service,
- misrepresenting provider of service,
- waiving of deductibles or copays,
- Incorrect reporting of diagnoses or procedures (includes unbundling),
- overutilization of services,
- corruption (kickbacks and bribery),
- false or unnecessary issuance of prescription drugs.

Source: (Piper, 2013)

The sixth item in the list above may seem strange. Why is waiving your deductible or copay considered fraud? Many providers do not understand why they cannot choose to give a break to a particular patient. The reason is, in the eyes of the insurer, if the provider is willing to give a discount to one person, then they are over-charging everyone else for those same services. Consider this example.

- A provider's nephew (Bob) comes to see him and the provider performs a service that normally costs $100.

- According to Bob's plan, Bob should pay a twenty-dollar copay, and the remaining eighty-dollars should be paid by the insurer, and the provider collects a total of $100.

- If the provider waives Bob's copay, then Bob pays nothing, and the insurer pays eighty-dollars. The provider collects only eighty-dollars total for that service. Thus, effectively charging Bob less for the same service, which in this case is acceptable in the provider's eyes because Bob is a family member.

- If the insurer is aware of this, they will feel that the provider is willing to accept eighty-dollars for that service, and they should only really need to be paying sixty dollars instead of eighty.

- By charging other patients the full $100, they are stealing money from the insurer and committing fraud.

There are some ways to waive certain charges to other healthcare professionals as a professional courtesy and to patients with documented hardships, but the best thing to do is avoid this practice altogether unless there are clearly documented procedures ensuring that the discount is applied consistently.

The FBI's website contains press releases regarding health insurance fraud schemes that have been thwarted, or cases where arrests have been made. To illustrate the seriousness of healthcare fraud in this country, here are a few examples taken from press releases on the FBI's web site that have occurred in just one month. These are all from October 2019 which saw thirty-eight FBI press releases related to health insurance fraud cases. The cases listed below are only a fraction of the cases for that month:

- October 3: "Four People Charged, Fifth Pleads Guilty, in $4.5 Million Fraud Conspiracy Targeting State Health Benefits Programs"
- October 7: "Texas Physician Convicted in $16 Million Medicare Fraud Scheme"
- October 10: "Registered Nurse Indicted for HealthCare Fraud"
- October 18: "Long Island Chiropractor Sentenced to 18 Months' Imprisonment for Multi-Million-Dollar HealthCare Fraud Scheme"
- October 24: "Thirteen Convicted in $189 Million Medicare Kickback Scheme"
- October 29: "Man Sentenced for Stealing More Than $300,000 as Part of a Healthcare Fraud Scheme"
Source: (FBI.gov, 2019)

You can see that this is a wide-spread problem despite the severe consequences if they are caught. And healthcare fraud sometimes has effects on society far beyond insurance premiums.   Healthcare insurance fraud often puts people in physical danger by committing unnecessary medical procedures. Consider this example obtained from the National HealthCare Anti-fraud Association's website:

- In December, 2015, an Ohio cardiologist was sentenced to 20 years in federal prison for performing unnecessary catheterizations, tests, stent insertions and causing unnecessary coronary artery bypass surgeries as part of a scheme to overbill Medicare and other insurers by $29 million.

Source: (NHCAA.org, 2020)

It's not only providers and other healthcare-professionals who commit health insurance fraud. It is sometimes also committed by the consumer. By *knowingly providing false information* to an insurer for the purpose of having the insurer make payments to you or on your behalf, you are committing fraud. The following items are considered consumer health insurance fraud:

- Using a false or expired identification card to obtain treatment or medication

- Lending a medical identification card to a person who is not covered under your health insurance plan

- Adding someone to your health insurance plan who is not eligible (such as an ex-spouse or grandchildren)

- Forging or altering medical bills or receipts

- Submitting claims for services that you did not receive

CHAPTER 19

Regulation

The federal government recognizes the importance of health insurance to American society, and as such, the government protects consumers from unfair practices. This chapter provides a high-level look at how the health insurance industry is regulated.

The majority of regulation in the health insurance industry is from the individual states' legislatures and insurance oversight departments.

> *State regulation of insurance actually began in the nineteenth century when the state of New Hampshire appointed the very first insurance commissioner in 1851. As the industry evolved, so did the regulations.*

In 1945, the seventy-ninth Congress passed the McCarran–Ferguson Act, which provides that even though health insurance may be national in scope, the regulation of insurance should be left to the states. Because of this law, in general, the business of insurance is exempt from most federal regulation, including federal antitrust laws.

The method of regulation varies from state-to-sate. However, the National Association of Insurance Commissioners (NAIC) is the U.S. standard-setting and regulatory support organization created and governed by the chief insurance regulators from the fifty states, the District of Columbia, and five U.S. territories. The NAIC provides some semblance of consistency between the states.

In addition to the McCarran-Ferguson Act at the federal level, there are a few other federal laws that are applicable to health insurance. They include the Health Insurance Portability and Accountability Act, Consolidated Omnibus Budget Reconciliation Act, the Employee Retirement Income Security Act of 1974, and now the Affordable Care Act. Each of the laws mentioned above is described throughout this guide.

Every state passes state laws, and has state government insurance agencies to protect consumers from unfair health insurance practices. But most self-funded private sector health insurance plans are governed by the laws of ERISA, and are not subject to state regulations. ERISA itself requires "self-insured" plans to be regulated *only* at the federal level because there is no actual insurance company involved. Insurance companied offering fully-insured health insurance plans remain subject to insurance regulations at the state level. So ERISA is one of the major regulatory authorities for self-insured health insurance plans. The Department of Labor (DOL) enforces most of ERISA's provisions, and violating ERISA rules can have serious and costly consequences.

Primarily, there are only two types of employers that are exempt from ERISA requirements and regulation:

- Employee benefit plans maintained by federal, state, or local government

- Church plans established or maintained by a church or by a convention or association of churches

The regulations in ERISA have been the subject of many lawsuits because of conflicts created between federal and state law and each of their regulatory authority. This has gotten even more attention since the Affordable Care Act was enacted in 2010, with some cases reaching the U.S. Supreme Court.

CHAPTER 20

The Affordable Care Act (Obamacare)

The most significant thing that has occurred in health insurance regulation during the twenty-first century has been the adoption of the Affordable Care Act. It is important that you understand what the act is, why it has been enacted, and why it is the subject of intense political debate. It is helpful to have all the background from previous chapters before discussing the ACA.

The official name for the act that has been signed into law in 2010 is the Patient Protection and Affordable Care Act. It is often abbreviated as PPACA or simply ACA. It is also often referred to as Obamacare because it is a healthcare reform law signed by then president Barack Obama and introduced by Democrats during his administration. It has been a major overhaul of the U.S. healthcare system, and aimed to reduce the amount of money the average U.S. family paid for healthcare and ensure that more Americans have some kind of healthcare. One of the major requirements of the ACA is requiring everyone in the United States to have health insurance or pay a penalty. Some of the law's provisions started immediately, most of the major ones have gone into effect in 2014, and the rest continue to roll out until 2022.

In previous chapters, you have seen some examples of how expensive healthcare can be. You have also learned that people who have health insurance can rest just a little bit easier knowing that should anything happen to them, the insurance will pay a portion or majority of the bills. But before 2010, many people did not have health insurance. Some estimates say there were between forty and fifty million people in the United States without health insurance. If you are employed, there is a good chance that you are offered health insurance by your employer. But some jobs and smaller employers have not offered health insurance to their employees, and even if they have, there has been no requirement to enroll. You could purchase private health insurance, which is very expensive, but most people would rather take a chance than pay the high premiums. They were willing to accept the risk. And if they had some kind of chronic condition (called pre-existing condition), most insurance companies would not even cover them or would charge even higher premiums for coverage.

People without insurance who need medical care will often simply not pay their bills. We all know how unpaid bills can affect a person and their family personally. But the large-scale problem is that this has been adding even more cost to the already out-of-control cost of healthcare because those unpaid charges have to be offset somewhere.

Obamacare, or the ACA required people to obtain health insurance, or pay a special tax (individual mandate), sometimes referred to as a penalty, and sometimes a tax. Threatening people with a financial penalty if they did not obtain health insurance was not going to be enough, so the ACA aimed to make it less expensive for people to obtain health insurance in the hopes that this would further incentivize people who didn't have insurance due to the cost. The ACA created exchanges, run by the federal government or state governments where people can shop for affordable health insurance and compare plans. A large part of

Obamacare has involved providing significant subsidies for lower-income people to help them afford the cost of health insurance, as well as expanding the eligibility for Medicare subsidies to make them available to more people.

The law is rather long and contains a number of things that are related to improving the healthcare system in the United States, making people healthier, and reducing costs. The law itself was over 2300 pages when it was signed, but has changed continuously since then. But, if someone asks you to explain Obamacare in a few sentences, you might summarize it in this way:

- Provide subsidies to lower income people so they can afford health insurance

- Require everyone to have health insurance or pay a penalty

- Make health insurance more affordable in general, and as a result everyone (or at least more or most people) will have health insurance

The ACA has established something called minimum essential coverage (MEC). This has established the level of coverage that a person needs to obtain to avoid the individual mandate penalty. The ACA also requires that all health insurance plans include certain benefits and that the insurer has to pay for certain preventative services completely. It also says insurers *cannot* turn you down or charge you more if you have a pre-existing condition.

When most people think of Obamacare there are a few things that typically come to mind. This is because there are certain details that are more likely to affect the average consumer of healthcare. Some of the important protections of ACA are as follows:

- It requires insurance plans to cover people with pre-existing health conditions, including pregnancy, without charging more,

- It provides free preventive care,

- It gives young adults more coverage options,

- It ends lifetime and yearly dollar limits on coverage of essential health benefits,

- It helps you understand the coverage you're getting,

- It makes it illegal for health insurance companies to cancel your health insurance just because you get sick.

Source: (HealthCare.gov Affordable Care Act (ACA), 2020)

Individual Mandate:

A major premise of the ACA is that, by requiring everyone to have health insurance, the healthy people will partially pay for the sick people. The young will pay for the old. Depending on your political views, this makes perfect sense. And when you think about it, it isn't much different from being required to have automobile insurance. It is a requirement under the law that everyone (who drives) has a certain level of automobile insurance. Those with clean driving records pay for those with poor driving records, and homeowners with no claims pay for people whose houses are damaged by storms. But your rates may increase if you have claims.

Many consider the ACA to be a form of socialism or representing socialist ideals. Defenders of the ACA, like ObamacareFacts.com, an independent site for ACA advice, argue that "[u]nder Obamacare we have a regulated private healthcare industry with a mix of public and private funding." It later goes on to say "A pure 'socialist' healthcare system would have total public funding and care (or would at least regulate every aspect of funding and care)."

There have been many legal challenges to the act and whether the individual mandate (or the entire ACA) is constitutional. The U.S. Supreme Court has ruled that the individual mandate was constitutional in 2012. But in December 2017 during the Donald Trump presidency, Congress passed the Tax Cuts and Jobs Act, which eliminated the individual mandate penalty effective January 1, 2019. And in December of 2019 the individual mandate was ruled unconstitutional by a panel of appellate judges. The argument then has become, if the mandate is central to the ACA, does that make the entire ACA unconstitutional? The case was returned to Judge O'Connor to determine whether the mandate can be severed from the rest of the law. Judge Reed O'Connor has ruled in federal district court in Fort Worth, Texas, that the ACA is unconstitutional because of how central the mandate is to the law.

Minimum Essential Coverage (MEC)

To be compliant with the ACA, health insurance plans must meet minimum essential coverage standards. Minimum essential coverage includes:

- Ambulatory patient services (outpatient services)

- Emergency services

- Hospitalization

- Maternity and newborn care

- Mental health and substance use disorder services, including behavioral health treatment

- Prescription drugs

- Rehabilitative and habilitative services and devices

- Laboratory services

- Preventive and wellness services and chronic disease management

- Pediatric services, including oral and vision care

Required benefits include outpatient care coverage, hospitalization, rehabilitative services and preventative care. Newborn, pediatric and maternity care also fall under this umbrella.

Source: (HealthCare.gov, 2020)

Employer Mandate

Under the ACA, employers must offer health insurance that is affordable and provides minimum value to ninety-five percent of their full-time employees and their children up to age twenty-six, or be subject to penalties. This is known as the employer mandate. It applies to employers with fifty or more full-time employees (employees who work thirty or more hours per week).

Small employers with less than fifty full-time employees are not subject to the employer mandate. Thus, they need not provide their employees with health insurance coverage. However, small employers who do provide their employees with health insurance may qualify for the small business healthcare tax credit. This credit is equal to one-half of the premiums small employers pay for their employees' health insurance. The tax credit is available to eligible employers for two consecutive tax years.

> *An unintended consequence of the ACA was that some people lost health insurance coverage offered through their employer. Some employers realized that it was less expensive to pay the penalties than to pay the insurance premiums for employees. This forced some people to have to shop for insurance for themselves and their families on the healthcare marketplace at a higher overall cost.*

Essential Health Benefits (EHBs)

Under the ACA, most health insurance plans are required to cover certain preventive services without cost to you, including the following.

Adults

- Abdominal aortic aneurysm screening: one-time for men of specified ages who have ever smoked
- Aspirin use to prevent cardiovascular disease for men and women of certain ages
- Blood pressure screening

- Cholesterol screening for adults of certain ages or at higher risk
- Colorectal cancer screening for adults over fifty
- Depression screening
- Diabetes (type 2) screening for adults with high blood pressure
- Certain immunizations for adults, such as the flu shot

Women

- Anemia screening routinely for pregnant women or women who may become pregnant
- Breastfeeding comprehensive support and counseling from trained providers, and access to breastfeeding supplies, for pregnant and nursing women
- FDA-approved contraceptive methods, sterilization procedures, and patient education and counseling, as prescribed by a healthcare provider for women with reproductive capacity (not including abortifacient drugs). This does not apply to health plans sponsored by certain exempt "religious employers."
- Breast cancer mammography screenings every one to two years for women over forty
- Cervical cancer screening for sexually active women
- Osteoporosis screening for women over age sixty depending on risk factors
- Well-woman visits to get recommended services for women under sixty-five

Children

- Autism screening for children at eighteen and twenty-four months
- Behavioral assessments
- Blood pressure screening
- Depression screening for adolescents
- Developmental screening for children under age three
- Hearing screening for all newborns

- Vaccines for illnesses such as whooping cough, influenza and chickenpox

Source: (HealthCare.gov, 2020)

Marketplace:

The health insurance marketplace was established by the ACA as a website that offers health insurance plans to individuals, families or small businesses. The health insurance plans offered on the marketplace are created and managed by private insurance companies, not the federal government. However, the health insurance plans that are sold on the marketplace are fully compliant with ACA requirements. The federal government runs and pays for the website where the plans are offered and sold. The ACA established the marketplace to make it easier for people to obtain health insurance in the hopes of increasing compliance with the individual mandate. Many states offer their own marketplace websites while the federal government manages a website (HealthCare.gov) open to residents of states that do not offer their own. Individuals can compare and apply for plans in the Marketplace during an open enrollment period each year. Like other health insurance plans, the plans sold on the marketplace have a special enrollment period that you may qualify for if you have certain life events such as getting married, having a baby, or losing health coverage.

> *It is difficult to know how much it actually cost to create the federal marketplace, including the website HealthCare.gov, because contracts are bundled, and it depends on what work you include in the estimate. But conservative estimates put the price-tag at seventy Million Dollars, and it was full of problems when it was initially rolled out to the public.*

Grandfathered plans

Health insurance plans that were in place before March 23, 2010, when the Affordable Care Act was signed into law, can be considered "grandfathered". These plans are allowed to offer the coverage they did before the Affordable Care Act went into effect even if they do not comply with the requirements set forth in the ACA. Plans may lose "grandfathered" status if they make certain significant changes that reduce benefits or increase costs at any time after March of 2010. Grandfathered plans are rarely seen anymore; however, some do still exist.

Effect of the ACA

After the ACA was passed, the number of Americans with health insurance benefits rose significantly. In fact, the number of uninsured Americans hit an all-time low, as you might expect, since there was a tax involved with not having health insurance, and the subsidies made it much cheaper to obtain health insurance. The implementation of the ACA was resulting in fewer uninsured Americans. This was a significant win for supporters of the ACA and its objectives. However, during the Trump administration there was constant banter about repealing the ACA or certain parts of it. And data suggests that after years of increasing coverage among Americans, the trend is starting to turn in the other direction.

Population of the United States without *health insurance for the entire year:*

2011: 48.6 million or 15.7%   *2012: 48.0 million or 15.4%*
2013: 41.8 million or 13.3%   *2014: 33.0 million or 10.4%*
2015: 29.0 million or 9.1%   *2016: 28.1 million or 8.8%*
2017: 25.6 million or 7.9%   *2018: 27.5 million or 8.5%*

Source: (Census.gov, 2018)

Having less uninsured people is better for the economy. Chapter 1 posed the question "Why do I need health insurance?" When people know they have health insurance coverage, they are more likely to see a provider proactively and less likely to avoid treatment of an illness that may turn into something much, larger in severity if left untreated. When more people have health insurance, providers write-off less unpaid charges, which strengthens their bottom line, allows them to charge less for services, and leads to lower medical costs for all. Having health insurance actually encourages healthier living and leads to less illness, a stronger economy, and better personal and financial situations.

LGBTQ

The ACA includes protections from many different discriminatory practices, such as increased rates for people with pre-existing conditions. The topics of gender identity, and LGBTQ rights have bounced around like ping-pong balls recently in many areas (e.g. the military, sports) including health insurance. Gender identity refers to an individual's concept of self as male, female, a blend of both or neither. Transgender then refers to those whose gender identity and/or expression is different from the sex they were assigned at birth.

According to the American Medical Association, approximately 1.4 million adults and 150,000 youth ages thirteen to seventeen in the United States identify as transgender. Many transgender people experience gender dysphoria which is a recognized medical condition defined by the APA as a "conflict between a person's physical or assigned gender and the gender with which he/she/they identify."

Every major medical association in the U.S. recognizes the medical necessity of transition-related care of transgender people and have called for health insurance coverage for treatment of gender dysphoria.

The ACA created specific protections barring insurance discrimination based on gender identity, or sexual orientation. Prior to the ACA, medically necessary gender-affirming hormones and surgeries were often excluded from insurance coverage.

In 2020, the Trump administration finalized a rule removing those protections. By defining "sex discrimination" to only mean discrimination for being female or male, nondiscrimination protections for LGBTQ people when it comes to healthcare and health insurance were removed. Under the new rule, a transgender person could be refused care for a checkup at a doctor's office, a transgender man could be denied treatment for ovarian cancer, or a hysterectomy may not be covered by an insurer, or may cost more. The courts were still debating this ruling when the Biden administration took over.

In 2021, the Biden administration reversed the Trump policy that sought to narrow the scope of legal rights of LGBTQ people involving medical care.

States passed their own rules, however if you remember from above, state insurance rules do not apply to self-insured benefit plans. Twenty states (CA, CT, CO, DE, HI, IL, MA, MD, MI, MN, NJ, NM, NV, NY, OR, PA, RI, VT and WA) and District of Columbia prohibit health insurers from excluding coverage for transgender health services.

LGBTQ people often forgo healthcare because they are afraid of being discriminated against. And just as with uninsured people, or people who avoid care because they do not understand their health insurance coverage, it could have serious or tragic medical consequences.

CHAPTER 21

COVID-19's Effect
on Health Insurance

It is both interesting and sad when I look back at the chapter on COVID-19 in the first edition of this guide. In March 2020, I wrote about 4,500 deaths throughout the world, 10,000 confirmed cases and almost one hundred deaths in the United States. By the end of March, the numbers in the United States were 300,000 confirmed cases and over 6,000 deaths. By mid-April we had 45,000 deaths with over 750,000 confirmed cases. That is the point where I stopped writing and the first edition was released in Mid-May 2020. At that point they were predicting the number of deaths in the United States could reach sixty to eighty thousand.

Unless you have been living in a cave, it will not surprise you to know that as we approached June 2021, the number of confirmed cases in the United States had reached over 32,800,000 with over 585,000 deaths according to the New York Times.

But there was good news; we had a vaccine. Two dose vaccines from Pfizer and Moderna were given emergency use authorization (EUA) by the FDA for those sixteen years of age and older in December 2020, and a single dose vaccine from Johnson & Johnson for those eighteen years of age and older received EUA in February 2021. The fact that vaccines were created to fight this virus in less than a year's time was remarkable. Normally a vaccine like this would take years to develop. But the president's Operation Warp Speed effort, and the fact that the research for this kind of vaccine had been underway for a number of years already made it possible.

After a slow start initially, by late April 2021, the United States was administering on average around three million shots per day. It slowed to around two million per day by late May. The slow start was the result of the logistics required to distribute vaccine across the country.

Low-income people; mostly minorities, did not have the same access to the vaccine as other people mainly because of their inability to go to where the vaccine was available. But that issue was recognized and addressed. In general, the demand for the vaccine was way higher than the supply. The Biden administration made distribution a priority. Administering the vaccine was left to the states. Some did it better than others. But the approach was to make sure those with the greatest risk have access to the vaccine first; those in nursing facilities and those over sixty-five years of age. At one-point teachers were given priority access to the vaccine so the schools could reopen, and slowly the vaccine was made available to more and more of the population. By April 2021, we had reached a point where supply and demand were leveling out, and the vaccine was available to anyone (sixteen and older) who wanted it.

Vaccinations were given free of charge to all Americans. As of late May 2021, the United States had administered over 250 million single doses of the vaccines with over 125 million people (38%) fully immunized against the virus. The United States was a world-leader in the administration of the vaccine as evidenced by the fact that less than ten percent of the world population had been vaccinated at that time. Drug trials continued to verify the vaccine's effectiveness (efficacy), and to make sure it can be given to younger people. By late May, it had been approved for children twelve years of age and older. More than 70 percent of Americans who were 65 or older were fully vaccinated, and 84 percent received at least one dose. Deaths due to COVID, hospitalizations and new cases were way down across the country. But the crisis was not over. Although there seemed to be extremely good results from the vaccines, there were concerns about the safety of the vaccines after a small number of people experienced side-effects. One to five people per million experienced severe side-effects which equated to .0001 percent to .0005 percent. But this information only added to what is referred to as "vaccine hesitancy". There was a large portion of the population who did not want to take the vaccine. Either because they did not believe it was safe, they had deep distrust of the government and believed it is some kind of mind-control or tracking conspiracy, felt that it violated their rights to be forced to do anything, and those who remained loyal to former Pres. Donald Trump and believed his message during the latter part of 2020 was that the virus was a big hoax perpetrated by the Chinese to ruin the American economy.

The goal of the vaccination program was to reach herd-immunity. Herd-immunity is protection from an infectious disease that happens when a population is immune either through vaccination or immunity developed through previous infection. Scientists believed we would reach herd-immunity when around eighty percent of the population was immunized. Because of vaccine hesitancy, it was not clear if we could ever reach that goal. Also, the vaccines were created to fight the virus as it was known in early 2020. Since then, it had continued to mutate, and scientists were able to identify different strains of the virus. So far, it seemed that the vaccine was effective against the strains identified at that time.

In March 2021, President Biden signed The American Rescue Plan Act of 2021, also called the COVID-19 Stimulus Package or American Rescue Plan into law. It was a $1.9 trillion economic stimulus bill to speed up the United States' recovery from the economic and health effects of the COVID-19 pandemic and the ongoing recession. There were parts of the law that had impact on health insurance, such as subsidies to help people whose employment was affected by the virus, pay cobra premiums.

Things were however looking a little more like the "old-normal". Restaurants were opening (some close to full-capacity), sporting events were allowing fans to attend, and some events that were cancelled in 2020 were once again being planned and held. In May 2021, the CDC's guidance was that everyone should wear masks if they could not maintain social distancing. Those who had been vaccinated did not understand why they needed to wear masks, and there was discussion about what incentive people had to get vaccinated if they could not change their behaviors. In mid-May, the CDC modified its guidance to say that if you were vaccinated, you no longer needed to wear a mask outdoors or indoors.

But this guide is about health insurance, so I want to make sure the COVID-19 effect on health insurance is addressed. What follows is information that was presented in the first edition.

In December 2019, people in Wuhan China, (the capital city of Hubei province), began getting sick, some dying, from a strain of coronavirus that would become known as COVID-19. China began an in-depth containment campaign to stop the spread of the virus. However, by the time the rest of the world discovered that it was more than just China's problem, it had quickly spread globally.

At the end of January 2020, President Trump convened a special task-force to address the problem led by VP Mike Pence, which included the top infectious disease minds in the United States. To slow the spread of the virus, the task force recommended a strategy called "social distancing". Everybody was advised to remain at least six feet away from everyone else. Most gatherings of ten or more people were cancelled.

People who did not feel well were advised to stay home and away from other people as much as possible. Schools closed. States issued "stay-at-home" orders, declaring that people should only leave their homes for critical reasons. Restaurants, bars and any other non-essential businesses were ordered closed, unless people were able to work from home. The NBA, NHL and Major League Baseball all put their seasons on-hold indefinitely. Millions of people became unemployed overnight. The country wrestled with shortages of personal protective clothing, respirators, and testing supplies. The healthcare system became overloaded with sick and dying patients. The U.S. economy took a nose dive, and political battles ensued over how to obtain scarce medical items such as masks, face-shields and respirators.

To Slow the Spread, We Needed to Know the Spread

It became apparent early-on that the virus was spread from person-to-person, and that it was highly transmittable. To slow the spread, experts needed to know who was infected. Infected people (whether showing symptoms or not) needed to be quarantined. It became crucial to know how many cases there were, and a testing program was established. Testing became paramount. But several problems in the United States were going to affect the ability to isolate all infected people, and get accurate counts on the number of infected people.

We had many uninsured Americans before the virus first appeared, and now the number of uninsured people was about to double or triple with the number of unemployed. Among those who did have insurance, many could not afford the cost of testing, and for those who contracted the virus, the cost of treatment was expensive, costing thousands of dollars. The length of hospitalization for patients who had severe cases could be up to two to three weeks with treatment costs in the range of $20,000 - $30,000. The majority of which would be paid by insurance plans assuming in-network providers. For uninsured patients, the bills could be as much as $75,000. Something needed to be done to ensure that (1) those who were not feeling well were tested, and (2) those who tested positive were not fearful of high medical bills which kept them from seeking medical care. Health insurance became a regular topic of conversation.

Anyone who lost their health insurance due to COVID-19-related job loss was advised to look into COBRA coverage, or check if they had become eligible for federal subsidies on the federal or state marketplace, or had become eligible for Medicaid due to loss of income. One of the problems with Cobra was that it was a "continuation" of your coverage through your employer. Businesses were shut-down, some of them never to reopen again. Many employers were unable to continue health coverage for their employees without a revenue stream so COBRA was not an option.

Federal Response

On March 13, 2020, Pres. Donald Trump declared a national emergency freeing-up $50 billion in federal resources. Large insurance companies like Cigna and Humana announced that they were waiving copays for coronavirus testing. Other insurance providers followed-suit. Dealing with the large population of uninsured Americans became an issue, and people called for opening up the federal marketplace so that uninsured people could enroll outside the normal enrollment period. The Trump administration said no. Instead, the White House pledged "cash payments" to compensate hospitals that treat uninsured patients.

On March 18, 2020, Congress approved the Families First Coronavirus Response Act (FFCRA). FFCRA provided paid sick leave for full- and part-time employees who are affected by the virus. This act also established testing for COVID-19 as an essential health benefit (EHB). By doing that, it meant that testing must be covered by ACA compliant health insurance plans. FFCRA mandated. that all group health plans, whether fully insured or self-insured provide COVID-19 testing coverage (including associated visits to a healthcare provider, urgent care center or emergency room) without any cost sharing, prior authorization or other medical management requirements. This was a necessary move because as private insurance companies like Cigna and Humana said they would waive copays for COVID-19 testing, there was nothing requiring self-insured employers to do the same. Several groups called on employers to waive copays for COVID-19 testing, and encouraged them to offer telehealth services if that was not already part of their plans. By making COVID-19 testing an EHB, self-insured employer plans were now required to provide the testing with no charge to the employee. FFCRA also applied to grandfathered plans, self-insured plans that were previously exempt from ERISA requirements like churches and local governments, and Medicare.

Providing these "first-dollar benefits", as they are often referred to, would normally have disallowed a health insurance plan from being considered a high deductible health plan. However, the IRS issued Notice 2020-15 which stated in part, "[u]ntil further guidance is issued, a health plan that otherwise satisfies the requirements to be a high deductible health plan (HDHP) under section 223(c)(2)(A) of the Internal Revenue Code (Code) will not fail to be an HDHP under section 223(c)(2)(A) merely because the health plan provides health benefits associated with testing for and treatment of COVID-19 without a deductible".

On March 27, 2020, a three trillion-dollar economic stimulus package was signed into law, which provided many provisions related to health insurance. The stimulus package was called the Coronavirus Aid, Relief, and Economic Security (CARES) act. CARES addressed many health-insurance-related issues.

On March 11, 2021, President Biden signed the $1.9 trillion American Rescue Plan Act of 2021 (ARP) into law. The ARP is a comprehensive attempt to address problems raised by the COVID-19 pandemic and the accompanying economic disruption. One of the most important issues the epidemic has spotlighted is the fact that millions of Americans remain uninsured. The ARP addresses this in three ways: expanded funding for Medicaid and the Children's Health Insurance Program, COBRA (Consolidated Omnibus Budget Reconciliation Act of 1985) subsidies, and expanded subsidies for marketplace coverage, including for people receiving unemployment insurance. All provisions are temporary but may be made permanent or extended. The ARP makes major improvements in access to and affordability of health coverage through the Marketplace by increasing eligibility for financial assistance to help pay for Marketplace coverage.

The new law will lower premiums for most people who currently have a Marketplace health plan and expand access to financial assistance for more consumers.

State Insurance Regulators

Previously in the guide, you learned that fully-funded health insurance plans, sold and administered by private insurance companies, were regulated by the individual states' departments of insurance. The states' regulatory bodies began issuing directives for insurance companies. Some were requirements, and some were strong suggestions. But their goal was to protect the citizens of their states and ensure that testing was affordable and the costs of treatment if you contracted this virus would not create a terrible financial burden.

Some of the states that previously had not expanded Medicaid began seeking ways to expand eligibility to temporarily insure more of their residents, and many states created special enrollment periods for their state exchanges.

The state and federal governments either recommended or mandated the following:

- o   Removal of cost-sharing requirements for COVID-19 testing and treatment

- o   Removal of restrictions on early prescription refills to ensure that everyone had an adequate supply of their maintenance medication

- o   Extension or elimination of premium grace periods; policies were not to be cancelled due to non-payment of premiums

- o   Travel insurance policies that included healthcare expenses must include COVID-19-related expenses and the COVID-19 outbreak must be considered an acceptable reason for trip cancellation and trip interruption policies to be invoked

- o Expansion of home-healthcare services to help keep people at home

- o Elimination of cost-sharing requirements for use of telehealth services.

- o Removal of restrictions and penalties for the use of out-of-network providers

- o Removal of preauthorization requirements

- o Changes to the rules for HSAs, HRAs, and FSAs including

  - allowing enrollment, disenrollment, and changes to contribution amounts for health and dependent care FSAs

  - allowing reimbursement for over-the-counter drugs and medicines without a doctor's prescription and menstrual care products.

Medicare

As the pandemic unfolded, the Centers for Disease Control determined that older adults and people who had chronic medical conditions were at a higher risk for more serious COVID-19 illness. To illustrate that point, statistics in early April showed that about seventy-five percent of the COVID-19 related deaths were among people sixty-five years of age and older. This meant that most people with Medicare were at higher risk for contracting serious cases of COVID-19.

Medicare said on their website, Medicare.gov that their recipient's health, safety, and welfare in the face of the pandemic were their highest priority. And as-such, they announced the following:

- Medicare covers the lab tests for COVID-19. You pay no out-of-pocket costs.

- Medicare covers all medically necessary hospitalizations. This includes if you're diagnosed with COVID-19 and might otherwise have been discharged from the hospital after an inpatient stay, but instead you need to stay in the hospital under quarantine.

- At this time, there's no vaccine for COVID-19. However, if one becomes available, it will be covered by all Medicare prescription drug plans (Part D).

- If you have a Medicare Advantage plan, you have access to these same benefits. Medicare allows these plans to waive cost-sharing for COVID-19 lab tests.

- Medicare has temporarily expanded its coverage of telehealth services to help you have access from more places (including your home), with a wider range of communication tools (including smartphones), and to interact with a range of providers (such as doctors, nurse practitioners, clinical psychologists, and licensed clinical social workers). During this time, you will be able to receive a specific set of services through telehealth including evaluation and management visits (common office visits), mental health counseling and preventive health screenings without a copayment if you have original Medicare.

Source: (Medicare.gov, 2020)

We're All in This Together

The mantra "We're all in this together" was never as true as during the COVID-19 pandemic. It is likely that almost everyone on the planet Earth was affected in some way by the pandemic. Certainly, everyone in the United States was seriously affected.

Insurers were affect in the same way as others businesses. Although they were allowed to continue operations, telecommuting was strongly encouraged, which presented technical, as well as operational challenges. Even though insurance processing was considered critical infrastructure, companies wanted to protect the health of their employees and forced them to work remotely. Absenteeism also increased due to illness. While working with diminished resources, the volume of claims, customer service calls, and plan changes increased. Insurance companies declared business emergencies, pulled out their dusty business continuity plans and put them to use. Insurance companies were asked to continue to provide as many core insurance business functions as possible, but many states relaxed the processing time frame requirements for handling and settlement of claims.

Everyone began pulling together in their own way. Major insurers, whether mandated or not began announcing that they would waive all cost sharing for members receiving treatment for COVID-19. Cigna, Humana, Aetna, and Blue Cross all said they will waive out-of-pocket costs for patients who need treatment for COVID-19 or associated health complications. Many pharmacies began offering free home delivery for prescription medicine, encouraged the use of drive -throughs and began offering additional products for sale at their drive-through windows.

Long-Term Effects

The loosening of restrictions and waiving of costs were only temporary.   Some insurance companies and government agencies specified time periods for the rule changes, some were to be in effect as long as the national or state emergencies remained in effect, and some were completely open-ended.

It's impossible to know the long-term effect the COVID-19 virus will have on health insurance and the industry as a whole. At some point, our society— including health insurance rules—will return to normal. But we do not know when that will be or what the "new normal" will look like. It is almost a certainty that all or most of the above exceptions will be removed at some point. But we've been forced to completely change our way-of-life overnight. And some of the things that we have been forced to do *will* have long-term implications.

Take for instance telemedicine. Use of telehealth and virtual visits will become more common. Employers and employees are having forced exposure to telemedicine, and assuming they like it and see the benefits, its usage is sure to increase after the crisis. It may even change the business model of some physicians as they see the value in virtual office visits. Many providers hurried to build an infrastructure that allows them to support virtual visits. (Necessity *is* the mother of invention.) Now that they have utilized it, they may see more value in it and even feel it could boost revenue by allowing them to see more patients. They could set aside one or even two days a week for only virtual visits. It will surely change the way Americans view health insurance. Fear may actually decrease the number of uninsured Americans long after the crisis.

Part of the long-term impact is going to be due to what they call "long-haulers". Some people experience lingering health problems even when they have recovered from the acute phase of the illness. The reason for this is not known, nor is it known how long the effects may last or ultimately the severity. The National Institutes of Health refer to long-term COVID-19 symptoms as PASC, which stands for post-acute sequelae of SARS-CoV-2. More common terms are post-COVID syndrome, long COVID or long-term COVID. We do not have enough data at this time to completely understand, but lingering effects such as breathing problems, heart problems, kidney damage, neurologic problems, mental health issues, diabetes, and distorted sense of smell and taste are still occurring in some COVID survivors.

Definitions & Acronyms

A

administrator – The entity who processes claims, makes payments to providers and performs other administrative functions for a health plan.

Affordable Care Act (ACA)- A comprehensive law passed in 2010, aimed at reforming America's healthcare system to improve access and affordability for more Americans.

allowed amount or allowable - The highest amount the insurance plan will (pay) for a service.   When a network is involved, this is the negotiated discounted rate the provider is obligated to accept.

annual deductible phase (of Medicare Part D) – This is the first of four phases in Medicare Part D coverage. In this phase, you pay for your medicines and Medicare does not pay anything. Once you meet the deductible limit, you move to the next phase.

appeal – A formal review process that a claimant can request if their claim is denied by the insurer.   It could be internal or external review. It is mandated by ERISA and the ACA.

B

balance billing - If there is still a balance owed on a medical bill after your insurance company has paid everything it's obligated to pay, and the provider expects you to pay that balance, you're being balance billed.

benefits -The healthcare items or services covered by an insurance plan.

benefit period / benefit year - Defines the time when benefit maximums, deductibles and coinsurance limits reset to zero. It has a start and end date. It is often one calendar year for health insurance plans (January 1 through December 31) but can be any twelve-month continuous period.

bundled pricing model – A pricing model where a fixed price is estimated and charged for an entire course of treatment or "episode" such as heart surgery or joint replacement. Incentivizing providers to be efficient, lowers cost and increase quality of care.

BUCA – An abbreviation used to refer to the 4 major health insurance companies: Blue Cross, United Healthcare, Cigna, and Aetna

C

catastrophic coverage phase (of Medicare Part D) – This is the fourth and final phase of Medicare Part D coverage. It begins after the out-of-pocket maximum for medication is met. During this period, you pay significantly lower copays or coinsurance for your covered drugs for the remainder of the year.

certificate of insurance (COI) – In a fully-insured health insurance plan, it is a document that describes all the benefits, eligibility requirements, and exclusions of the plan.

Centers for Medicare and Medicaid services (CMS) - The federal agency that runs the Medicare program. In addition, CMS works with the states to run the Medicaid programs. CMS works to make sure that the beneficiaries in these programs are able to get high quality healthcare.

Children's Health Insurance Program (CHIP) – CHIP provides low-cost health coverage to children in families that earn too much money to qualify for Medicaid. In some states, CHIP covers pregnant women. Each state offers CHIP coverage, and works closely with its state Medicaid program.

claim / claim form - A form you or your doctor completes and submits to your health insurance administrator for processing and payment. It contains an itemized bill for services provided to a member, as well as codes to show the specific procedures performed.

claimant – The person who has received the medical services described on a claim.

COBRA - Consolidated Omnibus Budget Reconciliation Act of 1985. This federal act requires group healthcare insurance plans to allow employees and covered dependents to continue their group coverage for a stated period after a qualifying event that causes the loss of group health coverage.

coinsurance - A certain portion of allowable charges you must pay after you have met your deductible. Coinsurance is usually expressed as a percentage.

coordination of benefits (COB) – The process of determining if a person has other health insurance benefits, and coordinating the portion each insurance is responsible for paying.

copayment (copay) - The amount you pay to a healthcare provider at the time you receive services. You may have to pay a copay for each covered visit to your doctor, depending on your plan. Not all plans have a copay.

cost transparency - Making available to the public, information on the healthcare system's costs, quality, efficiency, and other consumers' experiences with care.

coverage gap phase (of Medicare Part D) - The phase immediately after the initial coverage phase. Not everyone will enter the coverage gap phase. In this stage, the plan is temporarily limited in how much it pays for your prescription medicine.

covered service - A healthcare provider's service or medical supplies covered by your health plan. Benefits will be given for these services based on your plan.

D

deductible - The amount you pay for your healthcare services before your health insurer begins to be responsible for a portion of the costs. Deductibles are based on your benefit period. The deductible resets at the beginning of the benefit period or when you enroll in a new plan.

denial – Refusal to pay a claim by the insurance company or administrator.

dependent - An eligible person, other than the member (generally a spouse or child), who has healthcare benefits under the member's policy.

diagnostic testing - An examination to identify a person's condition, disease or illness, or to test for the presence of a disease or illness.

Direct Primary Care (DPC) – A business model where people pay a monthly fee and receive personalized, free care from a provider. No insurance is billed for services.

discount – This is the difference between the amount a provider charges and the amount that they have agreed to accept under a network agreement.

donut hole – A Medicare Part D term. Another name for the coverage gap phase. This is a term many people use to define that period after the coinsurance limit has been reached. This is the phase immediately after the initial coverage phase.

E

effective date of coverage - The date your coverage begins. The effective date can also represent the date a change in your coverage takes effect.

employer mandate - The Affordable Care Act requires employers with fifty or more employees to provide health coverage to their employees and sets a minimum baseline of coverage and employer contributions. Employers who do not comply will face annual penalties based on the number of employees in the firm

Employee Assistance Program (EAP) – A program that offers free and confidential counseling and referrals to employees who have personal or work-related problems.

Employee Retirement Income Security Act of 1974 (ERISA) - A federal law that sets minimum standards for employee benefit plans maintained by private-sector employers.

essential health benefits (EHBs) - Benefits the ACA says must be included in every insurance plan. Most insurance plans you can choose from will include these essential health benefits meant to ensure that basic health concerns are covered. If a health insurance plan does not contain all of these benefits, then the plan *is not* ACA compliant.

exchange – Health insurance marketplace operated by a particular state instead of the federal government.

exclusions - Specific medical conditions or circumstances that are not covered under a health insurance plan.

Explanation of Benefits (EOB) - An EOB is created after a claim has been processed by your health insurance plan. It explains the actions taken on a claim such as the allowable charges, discounts, the benefit available, reasons for denying payment and the claims appeal process.

Explanation of Payment (EOP) – And EOP is a document sent to a provider after a claim is processed that explains any payment that is being made to the provider or why no payment is being made.

F

family coverage - Healthcare coverage for a primary policyholder, and their spouse, or other eligible dependents.

Federal Poverty Level (FPL) – A measure of income issued every year by the Department of Health and Human Services (HHS). Federal poverty levels are used to determine your eligibility for certain programs and benefits, including savings on marketplace health insurance, and eligibility for Medicaid and CHIP coverage.

fee-for-service – This is a health insurance payment model where a provider performs a service and creates a bill, and the insurance company or you pay for the service.

fee schedule – A list of allowable charges as determined by a network agreement or Medicare.

Flexible Spending Account (FSA) - An FSA is often set up through an employer plan. It lets you set aside pre-tax money for common medical costs and dependent care. FSA funds must be used by the end of the defined period.

fraud – Taking an action to obtain funds from an insurance company that the person committing the fraud is not entitled.

fully insured – In a fully insured arrangement, the employer pays a premium to an insurance company who then issues a policy and assumes the financial risk associated with payment of claims.

G

gap insurance – A gap plan helps fill the gaps left by traditional health insurance plans. It can help you manage deductibles, coinsurance, and copays. It is often coupled with low premium / high deductible plans.

grandfathered health plan – A health insurance plan in effect before the adoption of the ACA with no major changes since.

H

Health and Human Services Department (HHS) – A cabinet-level department of the U.S. government whose goal is the health and safety of the American people.

health insurance marketplace - A federal government website where you can shop, compare, and buy health insurance benefit plans offered by participating private health insurance companies in your area. You can access the marketplace via HealthCare.gov

Health Insurance Portability and Accountability Act of 1996 (HIPAA) - A federal law that outlines rules and requirements to protect your protected health information (PHI). Everyone who has access to PHI is required to follow HIPAA requirements.

HMO (Health Maintenance Organization) – A type of health insurance plan that offers healthcare services only with specific HMO providers. Under an HMO plan, you might have to choose a primary care physician. The PCP will refer you to other HMO specialists when needed. Services from providers outside the HMO plan are hardly ever covered except in emergencies.

Health Reimbursement Account (HRA) - An account that lets an employer set aside funds for healthcare costs. These funds are used to reimburse covered services paid for by employees. An HRA has tax benefits for employer and employees.

Health Savings Account (HSA) - An account that lets you save for future medical costs. Money put in the account is not subject to federal income tax when deposited or withdrawn. Funds can build up and be used year to year. They are not required to be spent in a single year. HSAs must be paired with certain high-deductible health insurance plans.

I

ID card (or insurance ID card) – A card that confirms your health insurance status, and summarizes important information about your health insurance plan. You usually provide your ID card to a provider before obtaining a medical service.

indemnity insurance - A fixed indemnity plan can help manage out-of-pocket expenses by paying fixed cash benefits paid directly to the policyholder.

individual mandate – The part of the Affordable Care Act that requires U.S. individuals and companies to provide health insurance for themselves and their employees or face penalties (repealed beginning with tax year 2019).

in-network – A provider who has a contractual agreement with a provider network. The provider has agreed to accept a discounted fee for services and your health insurance plan will pay a larger portion of the charges than if you have used an out-of-network provider.

insurer – The entity (insurance company or your employer) who is financially responsible for providing the reimbursement to providers for medical claims.

insured – The person whom an insurer has agreed to provide coverage for, often referred to as a member or subscriber.

L

lifetime limit - A cap on the total lifetime benefits you may get from your insurance company for certain conditions. A health plan may have a total lifetime dollar limit on benefits or limits on specific benefits, or a combination of the two. After a lifetime limit is reached, the insurance plan will no longer pay for covered services. Under the Affordable Care Act, lifetime limits are no longer allowed on essential health benefits, such as emergency services and hospital stays.

limited benefit insurance – A category of health insurance that limits the benefit you can receive regardless of the actual amount of the bills. It is often referred to as limited indemnity insurance.

M

marketplace – The health insurance marketplace (also known as the "marketplace" or "exchange") provides health plan shopping and enrollment services through websites, call centers, and in-person help. The federal government operates the marketplace, available at HealthCare.gov, for most states. Some states run their own marketplaces. It is also referred to as an "exchange".

medically necessary (or medical necessity) - Services, supplies or prescription drugs that are needed to diagnose or treat a medical condition as opposed to a convenience to the insured.

medical tourism – Traveling outside the United States to obtain healthcare

Medicare - A federal program for people aged sixty-five or older that pays for healthcare expenses.

Medicare Advantage – A Medicare plan that is administered by a private insurance company under the federal Medicare guidelines. It often contains more benefits than stand-alone Medicare.

Medicare approved amount - The amount of money that Medicare will reimburse a healthcare provider for a medical service or item.

Medicare beneficiary – Anyone who is eligible to receive Medicare benefits

Medicare participating provider - A provider who has agreed to always accept the Medicare approved amount for a service they provide. Medicare participating providers may not charge you more than Medicare's approved amount, even if they charge non-Medicare patients more for the service.

Medicare Part A – Medicare Part A pays for inpatient care in a hospital, skilled nursing facility care, inpatient care in a skilled nursing facility (not custodial or long-term care), hospice care, and home healthcare.

Medicare Part B – Medicare Part B pays for medically necessary services, (services or supplies that are needed to diagnose or treat your medical condition and that meet accepted standards of medical practice), and preventive services (healthcare to prevent illness like the flu or detect it at an early stage, when treatment is most likely to work best).

Medicare Part C – Another name for a Medicare Advantage plan.

Medicare Part D - Prescription drug coverage.   Medicare Part D plans are administered by private insurance companies either on their own or as part of a Medicare Advantage plan.

Medicaid - A healthcare program that helps low-income families pay for doctor visits, hospital stays, long-term medical, custodial care costs and more. Medicaid is a joint program, funded primarily by the federal government and run at the state level, where coverage and eligibility requirements may vary.

medigap – A health insurance plan designed to cover expenses that are not covered by Medicare.

Minimum Essential Coverage (MEC) - The type of health coverage you must maintain to meet the individual responsibility requirement under the Affordable Care Act.

N

negotiation – The process by which you or someone on your behalf tries to obtain a lower charge for a healthcare service.

network – A group of physicians, hospitals and other facilities that have signed a contract to be a member of the network, and have agreed to accept discounted prices set by the network for their services. It is also sometimes referred to as a PPO or preferred provider organization.

network provider/in-network provider - A healthcare provider who is part of a provider network.

non-network provider/out-of-network provider - A healthcare provider who is *not* part of a plan's network. Costs associated with out-of-network providers may be higher or not covered by your plan.

O

Obamacare – Another name for the Affordable Care Act (ACA). It is so named because the legislation was enacted during the Obama administration and is often associated with President Obama.

open enrollment period - The period set up to allow you to choose from available health insurance plans (usually once a year) or make changes to an existing plan.

original Medicare – Part A and Part B. It is so named because these were the two parts of Medicare that existed when Medicare was created in 1965.

out-of-network provider – see non-network provider

out-of-pocket (OOP) – Any charges that you incur that are not covered by your insurance and you pay from your own pocket. The most you have to pay for covered services in a plan year out of your own pocket is called the OOP maximum. After you spend this amount on deductibles, copays and coinsurance, your health plan pays one hundred percent of the costs of covered benefits.

P

pharmacy benefit manager (PBM) - A separate, or third-party, company that handles your health plan's pharmacy benefit. A PBM processes and pays for your prescription drug claims based on the terms of your pharmacy benefit.

PPO (preferred provider organization) - A type of insurance plan that offers more extensive coverage for the services of healthcare providers who are part of the plan's network, but still offers some coverage for providers who are not part of the plan's network. PPO plans generally offer more flexibility than HMO plans, but premiums tend to be higher.

preauthorization (precertification) - The process where members or their physician notifies the health plan in advance of treatment, (such as a hospital admission or a complex diagnostic test) to have medical necessity determined.

predetermination – A determination of benefits for a particular procedure or service before the service is performed.

pre-existing condition - A condition, disability or illness that you have been treated for before applying for new health insurance coverage.

prescription drug - Any medicine that may not be given without a prescription because of federal or state law.

premium (healthcare insurance premium) - Payments you make to your insurer to keep your coverage.

preventative (preventive) care services - Routine healthcare that includes screenings, check-ups, and patient counseling to prevent illnesses, diseases, or other health problems.

primary care physician (PCP) – The provider (usually a family doctor) who has been designated as the primary provider of routine medical care and healthcare management. The PCP is usually associated with an HMO plan. The PCP refers to specialists as needed.

protected health information (PHI) – Any information about a person's health, medical condition, or medical treatment that is protected under the rules of HIPAA.

provider (or healthcare provider) - A hospital, facility, physician or other licensed healthcare professional who provides medical services.

Q

qualifying event – In terms of enrollment, a qualifying event is a circumstance that allows a person to make a change in their health insurance coverage when it is not open enrollment, such as the birth of a child. In COBRA, it is a circumstance that results in the loss of health insurance coverage, such as a job loss.

R

referral – Usually connected with an HMO or POS plan. It is a written authorization from a person's primary care physician to receive care from a different contracted doctor, specialist or facility.

Reference-based pricing (RBP) – A health insurance plan strategy where the insurer (employer) sets a limit on the amount it will allow for medical procedures. There is no network discount involved. The allowed amount in this case is based on what is determined to be "reasonable", and the provider is expected to accept it.

reinsurance (stoploss insurance) – Any entity who is financially responsible for paying insurance claims must protect themselves from large losses by purchasing reinsurance. The companies that sell this kind of product/service are called reinsurers.

repricing – The act of reviewing a claim, determining what network the provider is part of (if any) and letting the administrator know what the allowable charge is for the service(s) on the claim. They reprice the claim.

rider – A document that is attached to an insurance policy to add additional benefits, or modify the contents of the policy.

S

self-insurance (self-funded) – A method of providing employee health benefits where the employer assumes most of the financial risk of paying claims for their employees.

short-term insurance - A type of health insurance plan that provides benefits for a short period (six months or less).

specialist - A healthcare professional whose practice is limited to a certain branch of medicine, including specific procedures, age categories of patients, specific body systems or certain types of diseases.

subrogation – A process where an insurance company, administrator or third party investigates to determine who is responsible for paying medical expenses, such as a car accident or worker's compensation situation.

subsidy – Assistance provided to assist with the payment of health insurance premiums (typically) for people with incomes below certain levels. It could also be referred to as subsidized healthcare.

summary of benefits and coverage (SBC) – A document that summarizes a health insurance plan at a very high level. This is required by law.

summary plan description (SPD) – A document that summarizes a plan document. Sometimes a single SPD document serves as the plan document and SPD. It contains the plans eligibility requirements, benefits, exclusions, and much more.

T

telemedicine – A benefit that allows a person to call a telemedicine provider and speak to or video chat with a licensed doctor rather than physically visiting them.

third party administrator (TPA) – Also referred to as administrator. This is the organization that processes medical claims, and performs other administrative functions for a health insurance plan.

U

Utilization Review Accreditation Commission (URAC) – An independent, non-profit accreditation entity, based in Washington, DC, whose mission is helping promote healthcare quality through the accreditation of organizations involved in medical care services. URAC also offers education and measurement programs.

usual, customary, & reasonable (UCR) – The amount paid for a medical service in a geographic area based on what providers in the area usually charge for the same or similar medical service. The UCR amount sometimes is used to determine the allowed amount.

utilization management (UM) – The processing of determining medical necessity of a medical procedure or prescription drug. (preauthorization)

W

wellness – Activities designed to assist people with remaining in good health. Remaining Well. Such as exercise, eating well, getting the proper amount of sleep, and other healthy habits.

References

(2020). *29 CFR § 2560.503-1 - Claims procedure.*

ACPOnline.org. (2010, September). *Healthcare Transparency—Focus on Proce and Clinical Performance Information.* Retrieved from American College of Physicians: https://www.acponline.org/acp_policy/policies/healthcare_trans parency_2010.pdf

Amol S. Navathe, M. P. (2017). Cost of Joint Replacement Using Bundled Payment Models. *Journal of the AMerican Medical Association,* 177(2):214-222. doi:10.1001/jamainternmed.2016.8263.

Austin, T. (2017, September 5). *How Group Health Insurance Premiums Are Calculated and How You Can Manage Them blog.* Retrieved from GMS : https://www.groupmgmt.com/blog/post/2017/09/05/How-Group-Health-Insurance-Premiums-Are-Calculated-and-How-You-Can-Manage-Them.aspx

Batalova, J., Hanna, M., & Levesque, C. (2021, February 11). *Frequently Requested Statistics on Immigrants and Immigration in the United States.* Retrieved from Migration Policy Institute: https://www.migrationpolicy.org/article/frequently-requested-statistics-immigrants-and-immigration-united-states-2020#health-insurance

Bazar, E. (2017, November 16). *For Millions of Insured Americans, State Health Laws Don't Apply.* Retrieved from Kaiser Health News: https://khn.org/news/for-millions-of-insured-americans-state-health-laws-dont-apply/

Census.gov. (2018). *Health Insurance.* Retrieved from census.gov 3/31/20: https://www.census.gov/topics/health/health-insurance.html

Centers for Disease Control and Prevention. (n.d.). *Medical Tourism: Travel to Another Country for Medical Care*. Retrieved from wwwnc.cdc.gov: https://wwwnc.cdc.gov/travel/page/medical-tourism

CMS.gov. (2018). *Medicare Part A and Part B Summary*. Retrieved from CMS.gov: https://www.cms.gov/files/document/2018-mdcr-summary-ab-1.pdf

CMS.gov. (2018). *Medicare Part D Utilization*. Retrieved from CMS.gov 4/2/20: https://www.cms.gov/files/document/2018-mdcr-utlzn-d-2.pdf

CMS.gov. (2019, November 19). *Fee Schedules - General Information*. Retrieved from CMS.gov: https://www.cms.gov/Medicare/Medicare-Fee-for-Service-Payment/FeeScheduleGenInfo

CMS.gov. (2020). *Advance Premium Tax Credit (APTC)*. Retrieved from healthcare.gov: https://www.healthcare.gov/glossary/advanced-premium-tax-credit/

CMS.gov. (2020). *Appealing a health plan decision*. Retrieved from healthcare.gov March 2020: https://www.healthcare.gov/appeal-insurance-company-decision/internal-appeals/

CMS.gov. (2020, March). *Medicare Enrollment Dashboard*. Retrieved from Centers for Medicare and Medicaid Services: https://www.cms.gov/Research-Statistics-Data-and-Systems/Statistics-Trends-and-Reports/Dashboard/Medicare-Enrollment/Enrollment%20Dashboard.html

CMS.gov. (2020). *Official US Government Medicare Handbook*. Retrieved from Medicare.gov: https://www.medicare.gov/Pubs/pdf/10050-medicare-and-you.pdf

CMS.gov. (2020). *Your Guide to Medicare Prescription Drug Coverage*. Retrieved from Medicare.gov: https://www.medicare.gov/Pubs/pdf/11109-Your-Guide-to-Medicare-Prescrip-Drug-Cov.pdf

CMS.gov. (Page Last Modified: 03/24/2020). *NHE Fact Sheet.* Retrieved from Centers for Medicare and Medicaid Services: https://www.cms.gov/Research-Statistics-Data-and-Systems/Statistics-Trends-and-Reports/NationalHealthExpendData/NHE-Fact-Sheet

Committee on Health Care for Underserved Women. (2015). *Health Care for Unauthorized Immigrants, Committee Opinion #627.* Retrieved from ACOG.org: https://www.acog.org/clinical/clinical-guidance/committee-opinion/articles/2015/03/health-care-for-unauthorized-immigrants

Constantijn W.A. Panis PhD; Michael J. Brien PhD. (2019, January 7). *appendix to the Secretary's 2018 report to Congress on Self-fnded Health Plans.* Retrieved from US Dept of Labor: https://www.dol.gov/sites/dolgov/files/EBSA/researchers/statistics/retirement-bulletins/annual-report-on-self-insured-group-health-plans-2019-appendix-b.pdf

consumerfinance.gov. (2014, December). *Consumer credit reports:.* Retrieved from US Consumer Financial Protection Bureau: https://files.consumerfinance.gov/f/201412_cfpb_reports_consumer-credit-medical-and-non-medical-collections.pdf

Dmc.mn. (2021). *https://dmc.mn/what-is-dmc/.* Retrieved from Dmn.mn: https://dmc.mn/what-is-dmc/

Eves, C. (2020, August 10). *Germany: The New Frontier in Fighting Cancer.* Retrieved from cancerwellness.com: https://cancerwellness.com/travel/germany-medical-tourism/

FBI.gov. (2019, October). *Health Care Fraud News.* Retrieved from Federal Bureau of Investigation 03/30/20: https://www.fbi.gov/investigate/white-collar-crime/health-care-fraud/health-care-fraud-news

FBI.gov. (Retrieved 4/3/20). *Insurance Fraud (retrieved 3/31/20).* Retrieved from Federal Bureau of Investigation: https://www.fbi.gov/stats-services/publications/insurance-fraud

fda.gov. (2018, 01 25). *How to Buy Medicines Safely From an Online Pharmacy*. Retrieved from fda.gov 4/2/20: https://www.fda.gov/consumers/consumer-updates/how-buy-medicines-safely-online-pharmacy

FDA.gov. (2018, February 13). *Know Your Online Pharmacy*. Retrieved from US Food and Drug Administration: https://www.fda.gov/drugs/besaferx-know-your-online-pharmacy/media

GAO.gov. (2011, March). *Data on Private Health Insurance Denials (GAO-11-268)*. Retrieved from U.S. Government Accountability Office 3/31/20: https://www.gao.gov/new.items/d11268.pdf

GAO.gov. (2019, March). *Substantial Efforts Needed to Achieve Greater Progress on High-Risk Areas GAO-19-157SP*. Retrieved from United States Government Accountability Office: https://www.gao.gov/assets/700/697245.pdf

Goodman, J. C. (2018, 05 11). *High-Deductible Health Insurance: The Good, The Bad And The Ugly*. Retrieved from Forbes Magazine: https://www.forbes.com/sites/johngoodman/2018/05/11/high-deductible-health-insurance-the-good-the-bad-and-the-ugly/#62017b857b18

Gordon, D. (2021, Febuary 8). *Health Insurance Confusion Continues To Plague Americans, New Data Show*. Retrieved from Forbes.com: https://www.forbes.com/sites/debgordon/2021/02/08/health-insurance-confusion-continues-to-plague-americans-new-data-show/

Gorman, A. (2015, October 1). *Insurers Find Out-Of-Network Bills As Much As 1,400 Percent Higher*. Retrieved from Kaiser Health News: https://khn.org/news/insurers-find-out-of-network-bills-as-much-as-1400-percent-higher/

Government of Canada. (2017). *Healthcare in Canada*. Retrieved from canada.ca 4/10/20: https://www.canada.ca/en/immigration-refugees-citizenship/services/new-immigrants/new-life-canada/health-care-card.html

Grant, K. B. (2016, March 27). *It's Time to Get a Second Opinion Before Paying That Medical Bill*. Retrieved from nbcnews.com: https://www.nbcnews.com/business/consumer/its-time-get-second-opinion-paying-medical-bill-n545626

Hamel, L., Munana, C., & Brodie, M. (2019, May 2019). *Kaiser Family Foundation/LA Times Survey Of Adults With Employer-Sponsored Insurance*. Retrieved from Kaiser Foundation: https://www.kff.org/report-section/kaiser-family-foundation-la-times-survey-of-adults-with-employer-sponsored-insurance-executive-summary/

HealthCare.gov. (2020). *How to appeal a Marketplace decision*. Retrieved from healthcare.gov 4/2/20: https://www.healthcare.gov/marketplace-appeals/what-you-can-appeal/

HealthCare.gov. (2020). *Preventive health services*. Retrieved from HealthCare.gov 3/31/20: https://www.healthcare.gov/coverage/preventive-care-benefits/

HealthCare.gov. (2020). *What Marketplace health insurance plans cover*. Retrieved from HealthCare.gov 3/31/20: https://www.healthcare.gov/coverage/what-marketplace-plans-cover/

HealthCare.gov Affordable Care Act (ACA). (2020). Retrieved from HealthCare.gov 3/31/20: https://www.healthcare.gov/glossary/affordable-care-act/

HealthcareStaff. (2019, Dec 24). *We asked health execs for their 2020 wish lists. Here's what they said*. Retrieved from FierceHealthcare: https://www.fiercehealthcare.com/hospitals-health-systems/we-asked-health-execs-their-wish-list-for-2020-here-s-what-they-said

Healthgram.com. (2020). *Exploring reference-based pricing pros and cons*. Retrieved from Healthgram.com:

https://www.healthgram.com/insight/pros-and-cons-of-reference-based-pricing-health-plans/

HHS.gov. (2013). *Summary of the HIPAA Privacy Rule*. Retrieved from Dept of Health and Human Services: https://www.hhs.gov/hipaa/for-professionals/privacy/laws-regulations/index.html

HHS.gov. (2019, November 15). *Trump Administration Announces Historic Price Transparency Requirements to Increase Competition and Lower Healthcare Costs for All Americans*. Retrieved from HHS.gov 4/9/20: https://www.hhs.gov/about/news/2019/11/15/trump-administration-announces-historic-price-transparency-and-lower-healthcare-costs-for-all-americans.html

HHS.gov. (2020, 01 17). *Annual Update of the HHS Poverty Guidelines*. Retrieved from Federal Register: https://www.federalregister.gov/documents/2018/01/18/2018-00814/annual-update-of-the-hhs-poverty-guidelines

Hroncich, C. (2019, October 22). *A how-to guide for reference-based pricing*. Retrieved from Employee Benefit Advisor: https://www.employeebenefitadviser.com/news/a-guide-for-reference-based-pricing

Ireland, S. (2019, August 5). *Countries With The Best Health Care Systems, 2019*. Retrieved from ceoworld.biz: https://ceoworld.biz/2019/08/05/revealed-countries-with-the-best-health-care-systems-2019/

Julie Appleby; KHN. (2020, January 29). *A $41,212 Surgery Bill Compounded A Patient's Appendicitis Pain*. Retrieved from npr.org: https://www.npr.org/sections/health-shots/2020/01/29/800870904/a-41-212-surgery-bill-compounded-a-patients-appendicitis-pain

Julie Appleby; KHN. (2020, November 25). *A Kid, A Minor Bike Accident And A $19,000 Medical Bill*. Retrieved from NPR.org: https://www.npr.org/sections/health-shots/2020/11/25/937971995/a-kid-a-minor-bike-accident-and-a-19-000-medical-bill

Karen Pollitz, D. M. (2021, January 20). *Claims Denials and Appeals in ACA Marketplace Plans*. Retrieved from kff.org: https://www.kff.org/private-insurance/issue-brief/claims-denials-and-appeals-in-aca-marketplace-plans/#:~:text=In%202019%2C%20HealthCare.gov%20consumers,readily%20apparent%20from%20plan%20documents.

Keith, K. (2019, June 25). *Unpacking The Executive Order On Health Care Price Transparency And Quality*. Retrieved from healthaffairs.org: https://www.healthaffairs.org/do/10.1377/hblog20190625.974595/full/

Medicaid.gov. (2019). *December 2019 Medicaid & CHIP Enrollment Data Highlights*. Retrieved from Medicaid.gov 4/16/20.

Medical Tourism. (2019). Retrieved from MedicalTourism.com: MedicalTourism.com

medicaltourism.com/About Us. (2021). Retrieved from medicaltourism.com: https://www.medicaltourism.com/mta/about-us

Medicare.gov. (2020). *Medicare & Coronavirus*. Retrieved from The Official U.S. Government Site for Medicare 4/10/20: https://www.medicare.gov/medicare-coronavirus

medicare.gov. (2020). *Medicare Savings Programs*. Retrieved from medicare.gov 4/2/20: https://www.medicare.gov/your-medicare-costs/get-help-paying-costs/medicare-savings-programs

Menton, J. (2020, September 18). *'This is going to bankrupt me': Americans rack up $45B worth of medical debt in collections*. Retrieved from USAToday.com: https://www.usatoday.com/story/money/2020/09/18/unemployment-americans-face-45-b-worth-medical-debt-collections/3480192001/

Mobile Fact Sheet. (2019, June 12). Retrieved from Pew Research Center Internet & Technology: https://www.pewresearch.org/internet/fact-sheet/mobile/

NAIC. (2010, June 08). *Definitions for Health Accreditation.* Retrieved from NAIC.org: https://www.naic.org/documents/committees_b_consumer_infor mation_100706_urac_definitions_hca.pdf

National Conference of State Legislatures. (2019, March 29). *Snapshoit of US Immigfration 2019*. Retrieved from National Conference of State Legislatures: https://www.ncsl.org/research/immigration/snapshot-of-u-s-immigration-2017.aspx

New Model for Low-Cost High-Quality Healthcare: The Cayman Islands? (2014, October 28). Retrieved from healthcatalyst.com: https://www.healthcatalyst.com/news/new-model-for-low-cost-high-quality-healthcare-the-cayman-islands/

NHCAA.org. (2020). *The Challenge of Healthcare Fraud.* Retrieved from National Health Care anti Fraud Association: https://www.nhcaa.org/resources/health-care-anti-fraud-resources/the-challenge-of-health-care-fraud.aspx

Obamacarefacts.com. (2015 updated 2017, March 4). *Facts on Deaths Due to Lack of Health Insurance in US.* Retrieved from obamacarefacts.com: https://obamacarefacts.com/facts-on-deaths-due-to-lack-of-health-insurance-in-us/

Palosky, C. (2019, 02 25). *Analysis: Marketplace Plans Denied an Average of Nearly One in Five Claims in 2017 with Wide Variations across Insurers.* Retrieved from kkf.org: https://www.kff.org/private-insurance/press-release/analysis-marketplace-plans-denied-average-of-nearly-one-in-five-claims-in-2017-with-wide-variations-across-insurers/

Pianin, E. (2016, October 23). *Crackdown on Medicare Fraud Is Producing Some Impressive Results.* Retrieved from thefiscaltimes.com: http://www.thefiscaltimes.com/2016/10/23/Crackdown-Medicare-Fraud-Producing-Some-Impressive-Results

Piper, C. (2013, January/February). *10 popular health care provider fraud schemes.* Retrieved from Association of Certified Fraud Examiners: https://www.acfe.com/article.aspx?id=4294976280

Pollitz, K., Cox, C., & Fehr, R. (2019, 02 25). *Claims Denials and Appeals in ACA Marketplace Plans (Updated June 12th)*. Retrieved from kkf.org: https://www.kff.org/private-insurance/issue-brief/claims-denials-and-appeals-in-aca-marketplace-plans/

Richard J. Sagall, M. (2013, August 26). *Drug Discount Cards – Lifting the Veil of Secrecy*. Retrieved from CostsofCare.org: costsofcare.org/drug-discount-cards-liftin-the-veil-of-secrecy/

Sainato, M. (2020, January 7). *The Americans dying because they can't afford medical care*. Retrieved from theguardian.com: https://www.theguardian.com/us-news/2020/jan/07/americans-healthcare-medical-costs

SIIA. (2019). *Self Insured Group Health Plans.* Retrieved from SIIA.org: https://www.siia.org/i4a/pages/index.cfm?pageID=4546

Siwicki, B. (2016, August 5). *CEO Spotlight: American Well's Roy Schoenberg on the U.S. coming out of a 10 year telehealth war zone*. Retrieved from healthcareitnews.com: https://www.healthcareitnews.com/news/ceo-spotlight-american-wells-roy-schoenberg-us-coming-out-10-year-telehealth-war-zone

Stephano, R.-M. (n.d.). *Top 10 Medical Tourism Destinations in the World*. Retrieved from magazinbe.medicaltourism.com: https://www.magazine.medicaltourism.com/article/top-10-medical-tourism-destinations-world

Sultan, R. (2020, March 4). *5 Horror Stories About the Cost of Health Care Even WHen You Have Insurance*. Retrieved from Vice.com: https://www.vice.com/en/article/xgq5jw/surprise-medical-bill-stories-and-private-health-care-insurance

Team, M. H. (2017, 09 22). *2017 Survey of Physician Appointment Wait Times*. Retrieved from merritthawkins.com: https://www.merritthawkins.com/news-and-insights/thought-leadership/survey/survey-of-physician-appointment-wait-times/

Ungerleider, N. (2015, May 26). *The $6.5 Billion, 20-Year Plan To Transform An American City*. Retrieved from fastcompany.com: https://www.fastcompany.com/3041355/the-65-billion-20-year-plan-to-transform-an-american-city

USDOJ. (Retrieved 4/21/21). *Health Care Fraud Unit Facts and Statistics*. Retrieved from justice.gov: https://www.justice.gov/criminal-fraud/facts-statistics

Voigt, J. (2019, Fall/Winter). *Is Direct Primary Care a Viable Alternative?* Retrieved from Wharton Magazine Government/Healthcare: https://magazine.wharton.upenn.edu/digital/is-direct-primary-care-a-viable-alternativei/

What is Concierge Medicine? [Updated for 2020]. (2020). Retrieved from Concierge Medicine Today: https://conciergemedicinetoday.org/what-is-concierge-medicine-concierge-medicine-definition-concierge-medicine-defined/

Wong, V. (2019, January 17). *34 Devastating Stories About How People Are Still Crushed By Medical Debt*. Retrieved from Buzzfeednews.com: https://www.buzzfeednews.com/article/venessawong/34-heart-wrenching-stories-about-what-struggling-with

9 798734 716748